PSYCHOPATHOLOGY

PSYCHOPATHOLOGY
ITS DEVELOPMENT AND ITS
PLACE IN MEDICINE

by

BERNARD HART
M.D. (Lond.), F.R.C.P. (Lond.)

*Physician in Psychological Medicine, University
College Hospital, and Physician in Psychiatry,
National Hospital, Queen Square, London*

CAMBRIDGE
AT THE UNIVERSITY PRESS
1950

CAMBRIDGE
UNIVERSITY PRESS

University Printing House, Cambridge CB2 8BS, United Kingdom

Published in the United States of America by Cambridge University Press, New York

Cambridge University Press is part of the University of Cambridge.

It furthers the University's mission by disseminating knowledge in the pursuit of education, learning and research at the highest international levels of excellence.

www.cambridge.org
Information on this title: www.cambridge.org/9781107693647

© Cambridge University Press 1929

First edition 1927
Second edition 1929
First published 1929
Reprinted 1939, 1950
First paperback edition 2013

A catalogue record for this publication is available from the British Library

ISBN 978-1-107-69364-7 Paperback

PREFACE

THE major portion of this book is taken up by the Goulstonian Lectures on "The Development of Psychopathology and its Place in Medicine," which were delivered before the Royal College of Physicians of London in March 1926. These lectures endeavour to present a description of the development of psychopathology, and a critical review of the chief tenets held by the various schools of thought at the present day. Owing to the wide field included in this aim, and the limitations of space necessitated by its compression into three lectures, the subject has inevitably been treated in a summary fashion, and the views of many authorities have not received the consideration due to their importance. Certain topics, moreover, have been dealt with in the lectures in so brief a manner that the conclusions reached hardly appear to be justified by the evidence. In order to remedy this defect to some extent an appendix has been added to the second lecture, and two older papers have been reprinted in which such questions as the nature of suggestion, the methods of psychotherapy, and the value of evidence, have been considered at greater length. This plan has carried with it, however, the disadvantage that a certain amount of repetition and redundancy has been unavoidable.

The Goulstonian Lectures were originally published in the *Lancet*, "The Psychology of Rumour" and "The Methods of Psychotherapy" in the *Proceedings* of the Royal Society of Medicine. I am indebted to the Editors of these Journals for permission to reprint.

BERNARD HART

February, 1927

PREFACE TO SECOND EDITION

In the present edition no material alteration has been made in the body of the book. A new chapter on "The Conception of Dissociation" has been added, however, in which this conception has been considered at greater length than was possible in the Goulstonian Lectures. It is hoped that the addition will serve to amplify and make more intelligible the point of view which has been adopted in the Lectures with regard to the respective contributions to psychopathology of Janet and of Freud.

"The Conception of Dissociation" was originally published in the *British Journal of Medical Psychology*, and I am indebted to the Editor of that Journal for permission to reprint.

BERNARD HART

May, 1929

CONTENTS

THE
DEVELOPMENT OF PSYCHOPATHOLOGY
AND ITS PLACE IN MEDICINE

GOULSTONIAN LECTURES

I

During the past few decades psychology has emerged with disconcerting vigour from the paths of academic quietude, and has laid claim to a substantial share in the practical affairs of mankind. It has asserted its right to a place in the proud structure of the sciences, and its right to contribute to the understanding and control of the actual problems of human life. Among those problems is the causation and treatment of disease, and it is to the endeavours and achievements of psychology in this sphere that the present lectures are devoted. Our task will be to trace out the development of the psychological approach in medicine, to consider the scientific and medical value of the successive stages in that development, and finally to estimate the place in medicine to which the psychopathology of to-day is entitled. The justification of such a survey hardly requires demonstration. Interest in morbid psychology has increased immeasurably during the present century, and in recent years the literature dealing with the subject has been remarkable in its volume and variety. It is true that much of this has but little value from the standpoint of science, but some of it is solid work, and the claim is made that psychopathology has succeeded in elucidating, at any rate in large measure, the problem of the nature and causation of the psychoneuroses. Such a claim, relating as it does to a group of disorders which form a not inconsiderable portion of medical practice, clearly merits careful examination and appraisement.

Our task, then, is to describe the history of psychopathology as a branch of medicine, to evaluate its achievements, and to consider how far it has succeeded in establishing a secure position within the fold of science. As a preliminary measure it will be helpful to define the precise meaning of some of the terms in this statement of our aim, so that the extent and limitations of the path we desire to traverse may be clearly marked out.

"Psychopathology" connotes, not a mere description of mental symptoms, but an endeavour to *explain* disorder or certain disorders in terms of psychological processes. The distinction expressed here is of the greatest importance for a clear understanding of the subject. The description of mental symptoms constitutes clinical psychiatry, and is as distinct from psychopathology as clinical medicine is from pathology. In the former case we are concerned with the recording of clinical phenomena, in the latter with the elucidation of the processes responsible for those phenomena. To enumerate the delusions which a patient expresses is not psychopathology but clinical psychiatry, and we do not pass beyond this until we endeavour to explain the incidence of the delusions in terms of causal processes. Moreover, this explanation is only psychopathological if it is couched in the language of psychology, and built up of psychological conceptions. Drever has remarked that "the indirect explanation of experience in terms of nervous structure and nervous process is no psychological explanation at all, but a physiological one,"[1] and it is equally true that the explanation of morbid mental symptoms in terms of brain may be excellent pathology, but it is not psychopathology. How far it is possible and useful to explain disorder by means of psychological conceptions, or in other words how far psychopathology deserves a place in scientific medicine, is of course a legitimate question, and one which forms a chief subject of inquiry in these

[1] Drever, *Instinct in Man*, 2nd edition, 1921, p. 9.

lectures; but we cannot even begin to answer it unless it is clearly understood that psychopathology does not mean a physiological explanation of mental disorder, but a psychological explanation of disorder, whether that disorder is mental or physical in its manifestations. For example, an explanation of the intellectual enfeeblement of senile dementia, in terms of the lesions found in the brain, is a physiological interpretation, although the phenomena explained are mental in character, while an explanation of hysterical paralysis in terms of suggestion is psychopathological, although the phenomena explained are physical in character.

In the light of these considerations it will be understood that in the present lectures we are only indirectly concerned with clinical psychiatry, and that its history and development do not enter into our inquiry. It is noteworthy, indeed, that psychopathology has mainly grown, not from the study of insanity, but from the investigation of hysteria, in which the phenomena are in great part physical in their manifestations.

In the definition of psychopathology which has been given above, the word "explain" is used in the sense in which it constitutes the goal of scientific method. Karl Pearson, in his classical *Grammar of Science*[1], has analysed the fundamental features which distinguish science from all other attempts to deal with our experience, and the principles which he enunciates will serve as a standard whereby the claims of psychopathology can be tested and appraised. The essential character of science resides, not in the nature of the facts with which it deals, but in the method of attack which it employs. This method consists of three successive steps. Firstly the observation of phenomena, secondly the orderly arrangement and classification of the facts which have been observed, and thirdly the finding of "laws," which will serve to explain those facts, and enable us to predict and control the

[1] Karl Pearson, *The Grammar of Science*, 1892.

occurrence of future phenomena of the same order. For example, our knowledge of planetary motion evolved from the observation of the successive positions occupied by the planets, through the classification of those positions by Kepler whereby it became apparent that the planets moved in ellipses round the sun, to the construction of the law of gravity by Newton which explained in a single and comprehensive formula the track and relations of the planetary movements. A body of knowledge which has traversed only the first two steps has attained to the level of a descriptive science, but it is imperfect and inadequate until it has succeeded in passing on to the third step. This third step involves a transition from phenomena to concepts. The "laws" which it formulates are not phenomena which can be observed in nature, but are constructed by the human mind in order to account for those phenomena. They are, in other words, conceptual abstractions whose sole claim to validity is that they do explain the observed facts. It is to be noted, moreover, that these "laws" are not only conceptual in character, but are frequently built up of imagined entities which cannot possibly be observed, and may even involve qualities contradicting our general experience. For example, the phenomena of light are explained by the assumption of a weightless and frictionless ether, which not only cannot be observed, but is imagined to possess qualities differing from those shown by every substance which has been observed. This freedom from the trammels of phenomenal reality, which scientific conceptions claim to exercise, will be found to be a point of fundamental importance when we have to consider the justification of such psychopathological concepts as the "unconscious." It is necessary to remark that the freedom is only relative. Science does not entitle us to construct conceptions built entirely in the air, but only such as conform to the rigid procedure of its method. That is to say, they must explain the observed facts, they must not be contradicted by other facts, and they must be capable of verification by repeated reference to experience and experiment. The theory of light, for example, assumes an ether and the movement of its particles according to the laws of wave motion, but it only has scientific validity because every time we test our calculations by reference to experience and experiment we find that the phenomena observed are precisely what the theory would anticipate them to be. In other words, the validity of a scientific conception is measured by the service it is able to perform in the understanding, the prediction, and the control of the facts of our experience. So long as it can do these things it has a place in science, but when the advance of our knowledge shows it to be inadequate in these respects, or capable of being replaced by some wider and more satisfying conception, it is to be ruthlessly scrapped.

This digression to the basic principles of science has been necessary in order that we may have at our disposal a definite standard whereby to assess the history and achievement of psychopathology, and with this in our possession we may now pass on to the proper subject of our inquiry. The first task to be attempted will be a summary review of the history of medicine, with the object of discovering the beginnings of psychopathology, and the observations and conceptions which have served as the chief stones in its building. It may be said at once that psychopathology is a science of comparatively recent growth, and that hardly any traces of it are to be found before the middle of the nineteenth century. This may seem a strange statement in view of the prominent part played by apparently psychological procedures in medicine from the very dawn of history, and the oft-repeated assertion that psychotherapy is the oldest form of medical treatment. Nevertheless a perusal of the facts in the light of the general principles already laid down will show that it is substantially true, and that to regard the views and practices of early medicine as the first stages in the development of psychopathology is historically and logically false.

If we look back to ancient medicine we find everywhere the same essential picture, disease regarded as the work of demons or of magic, and a corresponding treatment by the aid of incantations, charms, and exorcisms. Side by side with these demonological conceptions and therapies, however, there existed a certain number of simple surgical practices, and a herbal lore in which one finds the names of drugs of undoubted efficacy and value. The Ebers papyrus (1550 B.C.)[1], for example, describes the incantations used in Egyptian medicine, but it also contains a list of remedies including such familiar drugs as opium, hyoscyamus, squills, and castor oil. The records of Babylonian medicine show a similar demonological view of the causation of disease, and detail the litanies and incantations necessary for its treatment. Diagnosis is closely connected with astrology, and is made by the interpretation of omens. "In the Old Testament disease is an expression of the wrath of God, to be removed only by moral reform, prayers and sacrifice."[2] Yet in both these cases there is ample evidence of the use of simple surgical, herbal, and hygienic measures, apparently without relation to the supernatural conceptions applied to disease in general. It is perhaps legitimate to assume that the former originally developed on a basis of empirical observation essentially identical with that on which the structure of science was ultimately to be erected.

Primitive tribes existing at the present day show in their medical practice features closely comparable to

[1] Garrison, *An Introduction to the History of Medicine*, 3rd edition, 1921, p. 49. I am heavily indebted to this invaluable work for a considerable number of the historical details contained in these lectures.

[2] Garrison, *op. cit.* pp. 54 ff.

those found everywhere in the medicine of antiquity. Disease is ascribed to the action of supernatural agents or of human magic, and treatment is carried out mainly by incantation, ceremonial, and exorcism, but again we find a number of remedial practices, apparently divorced from the demonological theory and therapy, and including the use of drugs and such measures as poulticing and blood-letting.

There is definite evidence that in these primitive tribes demonological procedures are actually efficacious, and that by their aid disease may in fact be caused and cured. Rivers remarks, "There can be no question that such processes as I have recorded here are efficacious. Men who have offended one whom they believe to have magical powers sicken, and even die, as the direct result of their belief; and if the process has not gone too far they will recover if they can be convinced that its spell has been removed. Similarly, one who has intruded on the haunt of a ghost or spirit will suffer, it may be, fatal illness, because he believes that he has lost his soul; and he will recover after the performance of rites to which he ascribes the power of restoring the lost soul to his body."[1] Now it is true that in the light of modern knowledge such results as these can only be explained by the invocation of suggestion or some similar psychological process. But, as Rivers later says, "It is necessary...to distinguish the production and treatment of disease by agencies acting through the mind from the knowledge that the measures used acted in this manner. Though remedies acting through the mind were probably the earliest to be employed by man, the knowledge that the remedies act in this way is one of the most recent acquirements of medicine."[2] In other words, the remedies were not given as a result of the application of a psychological conception, but either on account of their supposed physical effect

[1] Rivers, *Medicine, Magic, and Religion,* 1924, p. 50.
[2] Rivers, *op. cit.* p. 122.

or in accordance with a magico-religious conception. It is probable that many of the successful results achieved by drugs at the present day owe that success to factors of a psychological order, but their use has nothing to do with psychopathology, although the latter may ultimately seek to utilise the results as facts of observation. Psychopathology is a body of knowledge, and it does not begin to exist until an attempt is made to explain the phenomena of disease in terms of psychological processes and by the aid of psychological conceptions. Practically no trace of such an attempt can be found in ancient or primitive medicine. It is to be noted, moreover, that in early medicine demonological conceptions and procedures were applied to all forms of disease indiscriminately, and not merely to those conditions which we now class as the psychoneuroses and psychoses.

The demonological methods of ancient medicine, therefore, form no part of the foundations from which psychopathology has arisen, although the results they achieved can now be best explained by psychological conceptions. The roots of psychopathology must be sought for elsewhere, and they are to be found in the soil from which all scientific medicine has grown. The search for these roots will be facilitated by taking as a basis Rivers' statement that the beliefs of mankind concerning the causation of disease fall into three categories: (a) human agency (magic), (b) supernatural agency, (c) natural causes[1]. In primitive medicine, etiology and therapy are built almost exclusively on the first two, i.e. on magical and religious conceptions respectively. The category of natural causes hardly exists, but traces of it are nevertheless to be found in the domestic remedies and herbal lore which seem to have been employed everywhere side by side with the magical and religious practices.

It is this third category which contains science, although the latter is by no means coextensive with a mere belief

[1] Rivers, op. cit. p. 7.

in the efficacy of natural causes. We shall see that it is possible to hold many beliefs about "natural causes" which are certainly not cast in a scientific mould. Only with the gradual evolution of its peculiar method of attack did science succeed in building up a sharply defined body of knowledge within the general notion that disease was produced by natural causes rather than by magical or religious agencies. Now psychology and psychopathology are, or claim to be, branches of science, and therefore their development was only possible from the third category, and not at all from the other two. The failure to appreciate this necessary axiom was the cause of the long retardation of psychology in the advance of the sciences, and its trammelling with religion and ethics.

The magical and religious categories of primitive medicine frequently crop up throughout later history, dominating the picture in the middle ages, and occurring sporadically even in modern times, for example in Heinroth's doctrine that mental disorder is due to sin, and in the present-day conceptions of Christian Science. But they lie altogether outside the path of development of scientific medicine, and our only interest here is in the gradual evolution of the category of natural causes.

In Greek medicine we note the beginnings of what may be termed a philosophical approach to the problems of medicine. Empedocles (504–443 B.C.) introduced the doctrine of four elements (earth, air, fire, and water) as the fourfold root of all things, and conceived health as the result of their balance, and disease of their imbalance, in the human body. Later Greek writers postulated various other elements and qualities from whose combinations and permutations disorder could ensue, leading up to the "humoral pathology" embraced by Hippocrates, with its four essential humours—blood, phlegm, yellow bile, and black bile[1].

[1] Garrison, *op. cit.* pp. 80 ff.

In these theories of the Greeks we have an excellent example of a conception of disease which is certainly constructed within the category of natural causes, and is in no sense magical or religious, but which differs radically from the conceptions of science. It differs because it was not built up by the method of science. Scientific conceptions are imaginative constructions, but they must be erected on a solid basis of observed facts, and constantly tested by repeated descents from the plane of imaginative construction to that of experience and experiment. The Grecian theories are imaginative constructions built entirely in the air, and without any basis or control on the plane of observed facts.

Fortunately, at the same time, a certain amount of empirical knowledge began to accumulate, the direct descendant of the herbal and other simple remedial measures of older times, but immensely assisted by the development of clinical observation with Hippocrates. We know now that it was from this empirical knowledge that the structure of scientific medicine was ultimately to arise, and not at all from the proud but futile philosophical theories.

It is not necessary for our present purpose to trace out in detail the later history of the rise of scientific medicine. After the temporary submerging of all progress in the scholasticism and deductive mental exercises of the middle ages, medicine again began slowly to move forward. By the seventeenth century empirical knowledge had largely increased, and theories were developing which bore some relation to facts of observation, and gradually became more and more consistent with the method of science. These theories were constructed, however, of physical, physiological, and chemical conceptions; there was as yet hardly any indication of the birth of a psychological conception, and any germs of it detectable were generally hopelessly entangled with magico-religious conceptions. Here and there, however, we may note the sporadic appearance of a genuine psychological point of view in such writings as those of Henri de Mondeville (1260–1320), who in his surgical treatise counsels his readers to "keep up your patient's spirits by music of viols and ten-stringed psaltery, or by forged letters describing the death of his enemies, or by telling him that he has been elected to a bishopric, if a churchman,"[1] a piece of advice which is decidedly psychological, if its ethical standard is questionable.

The actual historical line of development of the psychological conception in medicine has its roots, though hardly its logical ancestry, in the seventeenth-century views and practices with regard to animal magnetism, and the personal power of healing. The ground for this statement is that, although none of these procedures were employed as the result of a psychological conception of disease or of therapy, and none of them form part of the actual building of psychopathology, yet they led to the observation of certain phenomena which were ultimately incorporated in the conception of suggestion, the conception which may be regarded as the foundation stone of modern psychopathology.

The notion that magnetism was a force capable of influencing the human body, and of being used for curative purposes, is found far back in the history of medicine, but it was in the seventeenth century that it became elaborated and systematised. In 1608 Rudolph Goclenius[2] wrote of the magnetic treatment of wounds, the general curative powers of magnetism were described by Athanasius Kircher in 1643[3], and in 1679 William Maxwell[4] produced a comprehensive account of magnetic therapy in which he propounded the theory that all

---

[1] Quoted by Garrison, *op. cit.* p. 146.
[2] Goclenius, *De magnetica curatione vulneris*, 1608.
[3] Kircher, *Magnes sive de arte magnetica*, 1643.
[4] Maxwell, *De medicina magnetica libri*, 1679, quoted by Janet, *Psychological Healing*, English translation, 1925, p. 30.

disease is due to the withdrawal of vital fluid from the
organs and can be remedied by restoring the necessary
magnetic force. The theory of animal magnetism was
therefore actually in existence long before the time of
Mesmer, although its origin is often erroneously ascribed
to him.

The personal power of healing is also a doctrine of
extreme antiquity, and records of its use may be traced
throughout history right down to the present day. The
power has generally been held to be the prerogative only
of certain persons, particularly royalty, and the "Royal
Touch" for the cure of diseases was frequently employed
by English and French sovereigns up to the reigns of
Queen Anne in this country and of Charles X in France[1].
In the seventeenth century the closely similar procedure
of treatment by "stroking" was carried out by less
exalted persons, and Valentine Greatrix, or Greatrakes,
acquired fame by the great number of cures which he
effected by this means. In a print in my possession he
is represented as treating a boy by stroking the patient's
head with his two hands, and is described as "famous
for curing several deseases and distempers by the stroak
of his hand only." One can hardly contemplate this print
and its legend without being reminded of the methods
employed later for the production of hypnosis, and the
place of such practices as a stage in the ultimate development of hypnotism and the conception of suggestion
cannot be doubted.

In 1766 Mesmer produced his thesis *De planetarum
influxu*, dealing with the influence of the planets on the
human body, an influence which he believed to be due
to a universal magnetic fluid. The distribution of this
fluid in the body, upon which depended health or disease,
could be altered by the will of another person, and cures
thereby effected. It will be observed that this theory is
substantially identical with that which had been proposed

[1] Crawfurd, *The King's Evil*, 1911.

by William Maxwell nearly a hundred years earlier. Mesmer attempted to put his ideas into practice in Vienna and various other towns, but it was not until his removal to Paris in 1778 that he began to achieve success. Here he opened a clinic in which he treated all kinds of diseases by "animal magnetism," under conditions in which it is difficult to avoid suspecting a considerable admixture of charlatanism with the sincerity which we may reasonably attribute to him. The patients were seated round a tub, the "baquet," containing various chemicals, and protruding iron rods which were applied to the portion of the body affected; the room was darkened, music was provided, and Mesmer appeared in a lilac robe, passing from one patient to another and touching them with his hands or with his wand[1]. Whatever we may think of Mesmer's methods there can be no doubt that results were produced, and during the following half century animal magnetism attained an immense vogue. Magnetic societies were founded in Paris and many other towns, several journals entirely devoted to the subject appeared, and a great number of books were published. Phenomena of this kind do not necessarily indicate that a movement has any solidity or value, as we have melancholy reason to know in our own time, but it must be remembered that many of the advocates and investigators of magnetism were men of undoubted ability, knowledge, and standing, and that these men were absolutely convinced that a discovery of the first importance had been made. The reason for this remarkable circumstance is that the observations upon which the magnetisers built their theories were actual facts, facts which could be repeated and tested indefinitely, and moreover facts which were new, or at any rate newly appreciated. The theories were no doubt fantastic, but the facts were sound, and it was upon these

[1] Janet, *Psychological Healing*, translated by E. and C. Paul, 1925, pp. 30 ff.

facts that the building of psychopathology ultimately began.

The facts observed by the magnetisers in the course of their investigations may be said to have included practically all those taken up or rediscovered by the hypnotists of a later age. Amongst these phenomena may be mentioned the production and removal, at the will of the magnetiser, of anaesthesias, paralyses, hallucinations, and somnambulisms, and the carrying out of what are now termed post-hypnotic suggestions, that is to say, the performance at some prescribed later time of an action commanded by the magnetiser during the magnetic state. The chief concern of the magnetisers was with therapeutics, but it is interesting to note that, although Mesmer and some of his followers applied their methods to all forms of disease, subsequent workers soon recognised that magnetic phenomena and curative results were best induced in neuropathic subjects. This circumstance indicates the first narrowing down to the definite path which ultimately led to the psychogenic conception of certain disorders.

The observations of the magnetisers were undoubtedly genuine and accurate, but they explained them by a theory which was already old, and which was certainly inadequate, the assumption of a magnetic fluid which passed between the operator and the patient. Teste[1], for example, explained suggested blindness for a particular object as due to the magnetic fluid being placed round the object in question and thereby rendering it invisible. Nevertheless the beginnings of a psychological conception were already apparent in the writings of the magnetisers. Janet[2] has pointed out that many of them distinguished clearly between the peculiar state (*état hypotaxique*) induced in the patient, and the actual suggestions (*phénomènes idéoplastiques*) which could be

[1] Teste, *Magnétisme expliqué*, 1845.
[2] Janet, *L'Automatisme Psychologique*, 4me édition, 1903, p. 143.

realised in that state. The magnetic fluid was invoked
by these writers to account for the former, but the latter
were explained in purely psychological terms. The distinction corresponds precisely to that existing between
the hypnotic state on the one hand, and the phenomena
of suggestion which can be observed while it is present
on the other hand, and it must be confessed that we are
still far from having achieved a satisfactory understanding
of the hypnotic state itself. It should be noted, moreover,
that the magnetic theory which sought to explain it is
not intrinsically absurd; the conception of animal magnetism is not in itself more fantastic than the assumption
of a weightless and frictionless ether to account for the
phenomena of light. Nevertheless it failed, because it
was not constructed according to the method of science,
and because it was found to be incompatible with many
of the facts subsequently provided by experience and
experiment.

Psychopathology has descended, not from the magnetic
theory, but from a reconsideration of the phenomena
observed during the magnetic state. The psychological
explanation of these, already foreshadowed in the works
of some of the earliest magnetisers, was made more
precise by Bertrand in France and by Braid in this
country, and with these writers the conception of suggestion may be said to have definitely arisen. Braid put
forward several theories in the course of his career,
veering round gradually from a conception of the facts
of mesmerism which was entirely physiological to one
which was essentially psychological. He showed that
the anaesthesias, paralyses, and other phenomena which
had been ascribed to the action of magnets, metals, and
peculiar passes, were due to none of these things, but
merely to the suggestive effect of the ideas aroused in
the patient's mind by the operator's words and gestures.
He reached the conclusion that "hypnotism," a word
first proposed by Braid as a substitute for the formerly

employed "Mesmerism," and the phenomena to be observed during the hypnotic state, were produced by
suggestion and to be explained by purely psychological
principles.

It is difficult to disentangle from the complicated
medical history of the first half of the nineteenth century
a decision as to whom the actual credit of priority in
this conception should be given. There can be no question
that many of the earlier French writers had foreshadowed
it, and the claims of Braid have been disputed[1]. It is
clear, at any rate, that with the publication of the latter's
Neurypnology in 1843 the conception of suggestion had
been definitely established. The formulation of this conception is the historical foundation stone of psychopathology. From it the whole structure can be traced,
including all the schools which at present hold the field.
Many of these schools diverged early from the simple
conception of suggestion along an independent road,
which will be subsequently considered in detail. For
the moment, however, our concern will be to describe
the later history of the concept of suggestion itself, and
to arrive at an estimate of its value and place in medicine.

The investigation of hypnotism languished after the
time of Braid, and it played but little part in medicine
until its resuscitation by the studies of Charcot and of
Bernheim in the eighties of last century. The place of
Charcot in this history provides a pathetic picture of
the irony of fate. A neurologist and a man of science,
with a keen appreciation of the necessity of exact clinical
observation and the establishment of objective facts, he
constructed, apparently by the very use of these accurate
methods, a body of doctrine which was even more false
than that of the magnetisers, and which subsequent re-

---

[1] G. Milne Bramwell, *Hypnotism, its history, practice and theory*,
3rd edition, 1913, and Janet, *Psychological Healing*, 1925, pp. 156 ff.
The latter work contains a valuable critical review of the history
of magnetism and hypnotism.

search has almost totally demolished. As a result of a
rigid investigation of the phenomena described by the
old magnetisers, carried out by himself and by his pupils
at the Salpêtrière, in particular Paul Richer, the author
of a monumental work on "grande hystérie,"[1] it was
concluded that hypnosis was a condition capable of
being produced purely by physical means; that it comprised three distinct stages, lethargy, catalepsy, and
somnambulism, each stage being initiated and terminated
by definite physical procedures, e.g. catalepsy by forcing
open the patient's eyes, somnambulism by rubbing the
head; that magnets and metals had a specific action in
causing and removing anaesthesias and other phenomena;
and that hypnosis was only found in association with
hysteria and was practically identical therewith. These
conclusions were based on the repeated examination of
a small number of patients, all hysterics, at the Salpêtrière. From the standpoint of our later knowledge
they afford an instructive and remarkable example of
the extent to which observations made with extreme care
and accuracy can be misapprehended and vitiated by the
adoption of too narrow an angle of approach. We know
now that the effective agents were not the magnets and
the physical procedures, but the words of the operator
and the expectations of the patient, that the three stages
were only an artificial result of the drilling and training
to which the patients had been subjected by constant
exhibitions and demonstrations, and that the physical
procedures which produced them could be replaced by a
word or any other agent in whose efficacy the patient
had implicit faith. It is true that Charcot was acquainted
with the conception of suggestion, but clearly he had no
adequate understanding of its extent and application,
and this fundamental omission was responsible for the
complete ruin of the structure so laboriously erected.

[1] Richer, *Études cliniques sur la grande hystérie*, 2me édition,
1885, pp. 505 ff.

We need hardly note that the work of the Salpêtrière school in the domain of hypnotism contributed but little to the building of psychopathology, although, as we shall see later, Charcot's investigation of hysteria played a much more important part.

The work of Bernheim, on the other hand, is in the direct line of the history we are endeavouring to follow. He owed his introduction to the study of hypnotism to Liébault, a practitioner who had for some years carried out hypnotic treatment in Nancy, but it may be said that essentially he repeated the observations of Braid, and arrived at conclusions practically identical with those of the latter, although amplified and extended in certain important directions. Bernheim's book[1], published in 1884, marked the appearance of a school of thought radically opposed to that of the Salpêtrière, and one which finally led to the complete overthrow of Charcot's views. The chief tenets of this school, the Nancy School as it is generally termed, are that all the phenomena observed by the old magnetisers, by the hypnotists, and by the Salpêtrière investigators, are the result of suggestion, and the hypnotic state only a condition of somnolence with increased suggestibility, itself produced entirely by suggestion. Hypnosis is not a pathological phenomenon, only to be found in hysterics, but a state which can be developed in the vast majority of normal people. Moreover suggestion is a universal factor in mental life, it can and does act in every one every day, and it can produce results, including therapeutic effects, without the intervention of hypnosis. Bernheim's wide conception of the place of suggestion has been aptly summarised by Milne Bramwell: "In other words, everyone is suggestible, and if you take some one and suggest to him to become more suggestible, that is hypnotism! Thus suggestion not only

[1] Bernheim, *De la suggestion dans l'état hypnotique et dans l'état de veille*, 1884.

excites the phenomena of hypnosis, but also explains them."[1]

We shall find later that there is ample ground for criticising the immensely extended part ascribed to suggestion by Bernheim, but we may pause here to note the marked effects which his view has exerted upon the subsequent development of psychological medicine. It has been responsible for a greatly increased recognition of the incidence and power of psychogenic factors in medical practice. This has been accompanied by the first clear appreciation of the suggestive character of many of the procedures of primitive medicine, and an understanding of at any rate one of the factors whereby those procedures attained success. Moreover, this viewpoint has been extended to the therapeutic practices of modern medicine, and has called attention to the necessity of differentiating the possible suggestive effects of drugs and other measures from any specific action which they may possess. On the other hand, it has led to a superficial use of the word suggestion as the explanation of all things psychological, and to an unfortunate tendency in the uninstructed to identify the entire spheres of psychopathology and psychotherapy with suggestion.

After Bernheim the historical development of suggestion has travelled along two roads which, although obviously closely connected with one another, have to some extent proceeded independently, the therapeutic and the etiological. That suggestive therapy should have marched along a road largely independent of etiological investigation is, indeed, a remarkable fact, and one which silently points to the inadequacy of such progress, but it is nevertheless true. Correlated with it is the further circumstance that the later writings on suggestive and hypnotic therapy show but little advance beyond the standpoint reached by Bernheim. Methods have been rendered more precise, and there has been a general

[1] Milne Bramwell, *op. cit.* p. 309.

though vague recognition that the methods are mainly applicable in certain types of disorder only, namely the psychoneuroses. Some of the writers have, moreover, concerned themselves with the mechanism of suggestion, but the general tendency has been to adopt suggestion as a kind of universal drug for the relief of symptoms, with scant investigation and discrimination of the causal processes responsible for those symptoms.

Bernheim's recognition of the fact that suggestion can be applied without hypnosis has produced a differentiation of methods into hypnotic and non-hypnotic, the latter comprising frank verbal suggestion in the waking state, and suggestion by what may be termed a "vehicle," that is to say, the deliberate use of electricity, drugs, or other measures, not for their specific effect, but as a means of introducing a suggestion into the patient's mind.

Throughout the history of suggestion the observation has frequently been made that results were sometimes apparently produced by ideas originating in the patient's mind and without the intervention of a second person, the term autosuggestion being finally evolved to indicate a process of this kind. This observation has in recent years become the basis of a school of therapy which, under the leadership of Coué and with the aid of the more or less systematic expositions of Baudoin[1] and other followers, has at the present time achieved a great vogue. Beyond, however, some interesting fresh formulations of familiar facts, this school does not seem to have contributed anything essentially new to our former knowledge.

It may be remarked that the waves of popularity which have marked the progress of mental therapy are an instructive object lesson. Animal magnetism rose to an immense vogue and fell, hypnotism has risen and

---

[1] Baudoin, *Suggestion and Autosuggestion*, English translation, 1920.

declined at least twice, Couéism and autosuggestion are at the apex of a wave to-day, and a closely allied surge may be seen in the astonishingly immense developments of Christian Science, New Thought, and other doctrines. It may be concluded that all these movements derive their temporary vitality from the undoubted fact that they do produce results, and therefore include somewhere within them principles of actual objective validity. We may call these principles faith and suggestion, but in this wide sense such terms are little more than a cloak for our ignorance. Whatever these principles may be it is clear that they are of vital concern to medicine, and it is the duty of medicine to dissect them out from their trappings, and allot them a defined place in our therapeutic armoury.

The second road along which the conception of suggestion has travelled concerns its application as a weapon of explanation in the causation of disorder. It was early perceived that suggestions were not only capable of removing symptoms, but also of producing them. Charcot, in his investigation of hysteria, came to the conclusion that certain of its phenomena were directly due to "ideas," an observation which, as we shall see, had an immense importance in directing the later development of psychopathology. Subsequent writers have endeavoured to show that these "ideas" were dependent, both in their origin and effect, upon the action of suggestion. This notion reached its full development in Babinski[1], for whom the whole clinical picture of hysteria was nothing but a manifestation of the results of suggestion. We may remark here that Babinski's view, though true enough as far as it goes, is so vague and superficial as to be of little service to our understanding of the complex problems of hysteria, but a more detailed examination of its validity must be postponed until we have

[1] Babinski et Froment, *Hystérie-Pithiatisme et troubles nerveux d'ordre réflexe*, 1917.

considered the position of the conception of suggestion as a whole. Suggestion is the first definite psychological conception which has been contributed to medicine, and it is therefore of fundamental importance that its nature and value should be accurately appraised. This problem cannot be attacked, however, until some general principles have been laid down to serve as a standard and test, and for this purpose it will be necessary to diverge for a moment from our direct path.

At the commencement of this lecture psychopathology was defined as an explanation of disorder by psychological conceptions, and it was pointed out that such an explanation must be sharply distinguished on the one hand from clinical psychiatry, and on the other hand from an interpretation of mental disorder by physiological conceptions. The question was left over, however, as to whether the explanation of disorder by psychological conceptions which psychopathology attempts is either possible, justifiable, or capable of forming a part of scientific knowledge. This question must now be taken up because, until it is answered, we have no sure ground from which suggestion and the later contributions of psychopathology to medicine can be judged.

The problem at issue is essentially a part of the wider problem as to whether psychology and interpretations in psychological terms have a right and a place in science. This claim was for a long time disputed, the opposition reaching its culmination in the materialistic philosophy of the nineteenth-century scientists, who held that psychology dealt with non-material and non-spatial processes which were "epiphenomenal" and "unreal," and therefore incapable of scientific treatment. Their view arose from two bases, the first being the unsatisfactory condition of the psychology of those days, for it was then an arm-chair production achieved by methods radically distinct from those which were proving so successful in the building of chemistry, physics, and other sciences;

while the second base was a total misapprehension of
the real nature of science. This misapprehension was
cleared away by the work of Karl Pearson and other
investigators, who, as we have seen, showed that science
is characterised, not by the nature of the facts with
which it deals, but by the method of its attack, and that
this method consists in the collection of facts, the classification of the facts collected, and finally the construction
of conceptions which serve to explain those facts. Clearly
there is nothing in this definition to exclude from the
field of science mental, as opposed to material, facts, nor
psychological as opposed to other conceptions. The sole
criterion which science demands is that the facts must
be rigidly observed, and the conceptions must be constructed according to the rules of scientific method. So
soon as these simple principles were grasped it was
obvious that psychology had a right to contribute its
quota to the scientific understanding of life and behaviour.

The behaviour of living organisms has been attacked
by several branches of science, each regarding the phenomena from its own standpoint, and interpreting them
in terms of its own concepts. Biology, for example,
interprets the phenomena in terms of life processes and
biological laws; physiology in terms of nervous energy,
reflex action, and so forth; chemistry in terms of the
interaction of chemical compounds. The essential point
which it is desired to emphasise is that there is not one
science of living organisms, but a number of different
methods of approach, each striving to deal with the
phenomena by the aid of its own concepts, and measur-
ing its success solely by the extent to which it achieves
the explanation and the control of those phenomena.
Psychology has established its claim to rank among
these methods of approach, and to attempt an explanation of the phenomena by psychological conceptions, just
as chemistry has a right to attempt an explanation by
chemical conceptions. Each of these various and more

or less independent methods of approach endeavours to attack as much of the field as it can, but it is found that while some of the phenomena are capable of explanation by the concepts of more than one branch of science, some can be more intelligibly and usefully explained by the concepts of one branch rather than by those of another, and some are at present capable of explanation by the concepts of one branch only. When the concepts of one branch are less comprehensive and widely applicable than those of another, there is always a hope that the former will ultimately be reduced to the latter. For example, we may reasonably anticipate that the concepts of nervous energy and reflex action will ultimately be reduced to the concepts of chemistry and physics. But such a reduction is mostly a goal of the future, and for the present each branch must be content to explain whatever phenomena it can in terms of its own concepts.

Now all these privileges and limitations appertain to psychology in the same measure as they appertain to the other branches of science which are attacking the problems of living organisms. Equally with the latter, psychology must be allowed to formulate its own concepts, and the value and validity of these must be tested solely by their capacity to explain and predict the phenomena, or, in other words, by what can be done by their aid. Again, we may look forward to a time when it may be possible to reduce the conceptions of psychology to the wider concepts of physiology, or the still wider concepts of chemistry and physics. But this desirable consummation is brought no nearer by the expedient of pretending it has been attained. There are many phenomena for which at the present time no other science than psychology can devise a feasible explanation, and many others in which psychological conceptions are more illuminating and helpful than physiological. We shall see that this statement applies to certain phenomena of disease, and so long as it holds we must gratefully accept

what assistance psychology is able to offer us, provided
the assistance is built up by a rigid application of the
method of science. It is not that a psychological explanation is right and a physiological explanation wrong,
it is merely that in certain spheres it is more profitable
to employ a psychological than a physiological conception. Similarly, if we talk of a disorder as psychogenic it
does not mean that no physiological, chemical, or physical
explanation will ultimately be possible, but only that
with our existing knowledge a psychological explanation
is more useful. In other words, a psychological conception
of a disorder may enable us to understand and treat
our patients, and if it does so it is sound science and
sound medicine, far sounder than the construction of
a quasi physiological hypothesis built altogether in the
air, without relation to any observed facts, and with
which it is possible to accomplish nothing. It would seem
almost unnecessary to labour these simple and obvious
facts, but the quaint notions of the Victorian philo-
sophers concerning the reality of nervous energy and
the futility of ideas are not entirely extinct even in the
medicine of to-day.

Armed with these general principles we may now
return from our digression into the philosophy of science,
and take up again the consideration of the conception
of suggestion. Clearly this conception is based on observed facts, and it enables us in some measure to explain
and to control the facts. Therefore, so far as its form is
concerned, it is validly constructed according to the
method of science and, as it is entirely couched in psychological terms, it is entitled to a place in psychopathology.
Its precise value, however, must be determined by a
consideration of the facts which it claims to interpret,
and its capacity to resume and explain those facts.

If we examine the phenomena for whose explanation
suggestion has been invoked, we find that these are extraordinarily numerous and diverse. When Bernheim

was developing his theory that the facts of animal magnetism and hypnotism were attributable to suggestion,
he made that conception so wide that Milne Bramwell
was constrained to remark, "In Bernheim's hands the
word 'suggestion' has acquired an entirely new signification, and differs only in name from the 'odylic' force of
the mesmerists. It has become mysterious and all-power-
ful, and is supposed to be capable, not only of evoking
and explaining all the phenomena of hypnotism, but also
of originating—nay, even of being the condition itself."[1]
Since those days the limits have been pushed wider still.
Babinski holds that suggestion is responsible for all the
phenomena of hysteria, other writers use it to explain
practically every symptom met with in the psychoneuroses. Others, again, maintain that all the methods
of psychotherapy, however diverse they may apparently
be, depend entirely for their effect upon the explicit or
implicit use of suggestion. Finally psychologists tell us
that suggestion is a normal process in the human mind,
and some believe that it explains our religious and political views, our caprices, and our prejudices. Now it is
plain that a causal principle which is invoked for the
interpretation of so many radically diverse phenomena
must be a factor so widespread and universally active
that it is a quite inadequate explanation of any particular
phenomenon. We may suspect, indeed, that for many
writers the word suggestion means little more than a
vague recognition that a certain phenomenon is to be
attributed to a psychological cause. Obviously, however,
if suggestion is to be a concept of value in science or in
medicine it must be brought within much narrower
limits than these; and in recent years many attempts
have been made to arrive at a definition marking off a
limited and homogeneous group of mental processes. It
cannot be said that any of these attempts has achieved
an entirely satisfactory result, but we have at least

[1] Milne Bramwell, *op. cit.* p. 337.

attained a more precise knowledge of the various processes which have been at one time or another subsumed
under the term "suggestion." Among these processes
are some, for example the simple communication of an
idea from one person to another, which are so general
and elementary that they have no value as part of a
limited concept. Another process, the influencing of
thought and action by the existence of emotional systems
which tend to inhibit ideas inimical to the goal of the
emotional system, and to enhance those in consonance
therewith, is so universal that it does not take us far in
the understanding of any particular phenomenon, unless
the precise nature and mode of action of the emotional
system involved is stated. It is this process that is no
doubt partly responsible for our politics, prejudices, and
indeed for much of our mental activity. Suggestion,
however it may be defined, is certainly to be regarded as
one of its manifestations, but unless the term can be
limited to a particular area of this very wide field it
cannot have much value as a weapon of explanation.
One possible limitation is to include in suggestion only
the process whereby an idea[1] which has been communicated from one person to another undergoes a further
development and realisation in the mind of the second
person, owing to the inhibition of all ideas which would
normally counteract it, this development and inhibition
being due to the existence of a peculiar affective relationship between the two persons. This sense would correspond to that in which the term is used to indicate a
particular therapeutic procedure carried out by a physician upon his patient, and it would include a considerable number of the phenomena commonly attributed to
suggestion in everyday life, but it would clearly not be

[1] The term "idea" has been deliberately employed in this
passage because of its conveniently elastic significance, though it
may be objected that it savours of an old and exploded psychological theory.

applicable to any and every process generated by an emotional system. Another possible limitation is to indicate by suggestion only the process whereby an idea undergoes development and realisation owing to the inhibition of counteracting ideas. This is of course a much wider concept than the last, because it does not specify that the force responsible for the inhibition arises from the affective relationship between two people, but permits of any force playing this part. It would therefore include autosuggestion, and the mechanism which Babinski conceives to be responsible for hysterical symptoms, as well as a great number of other phenomena, in fact practically all those which we have already characterised as the result of the working of an emotional system.

It is impossible here to enter into these complicated questions in detail[1], but enough has been said to show that suggestion is by no means the exact and definite conception which it is sometimes thought to be, and that it is used by writers in senses which are materially different both in their connotation and denotation. Probably the central kernel of all these various usages is the development and realisation of an idea owing to the inhibition of counteracting ideas by some affective force. This is undoubtedly a process of great practical importance, and a single term to indicate it would obviously be convenient. Processes of this kind are so universal, however, that their recognition will only give us a superficial understanding of any individual phenomenon unless we are in a position to go further, and can specify the affective force concerned, and the precise mechanism whereby certain particular ideas are developed while

[1] The nature of suggestion, and its function as an explanatory concept, are considered more fully in a paper by the author, entitled "The Methods of Psychotherapy," published in the *Proc. Roy. Soc. of Medicine*, 1918. This paper is reprinted in the present volume (see p. 125). A valuable review of the whole problem will also be found in Dr Ernest Jones' essay, "The Nature of Autosuggestion," *Brit. Journ. of Med. Psychol.* 1923.

others are inhibited. When Babinski tells us, for example,
that the symptoms of a hysterical patient are to be explained by suggestion, the statement is true enough if
suggestion is taken in the general sense which we have
described, but it leaves out almost everything worth
explaining—why this particular patient is so abnormally
suggestible, what is the particular emotional force responsible for the suggestion, and why he has developed
just these symptoms and not others.

We may conclude, therefore, that suggestion is a
legitimate psychopathological conception, provided that
it is used in one or other of the defined and limited senses
indicated, but that it only takes us one step towards
the solving of the problems we have to meet. This one
step, indeed, is of supreme importance, because it carries
with it the recognition of the psychogenic origin of certain
disorders, and implies all the significant changes in
medical theory and practice which must inevitably follow
from that recognition. Nevertheless, to regard suggestion
as a completely satisfying explanation of the clinical
picture presented by an individual patient would be as
futile as to regard the electric current proceeding from a
water-driven dynamo as completely explained by the
law of gravity. It is owing to this superficial character
of the conception they employ that the later history of
the suggestionist schools has been comparatively sterile.
They have developed some useful practical methods, but
in the understanding of patients and their illnesses they
have progressed but little beyond the standpoint of the
early hypnotists, or indeed of the early magnetisers.
For this understanding we must turn to schools whose
conceptions are more detailed and precise than that of
suggestion.

II

In the preceding lecture the development of psychopathology up to the formulation of the conception of suggestion was described, and an attempt was made to examine and evaluate this conception. We may now pass on to consider the history of a school of thought whose tenets are closely allied to those of the suggestionists. This is the so-called "Persuasionist school," and its chief protagonists in the literature are Dubois of Berne and Dejerine of Paris. Both are mainly concerned with therapy rather than with etiology, and etiology is with both authors regrettably vague and unsystematised, but they differ from one another in certain important respects. For Dubois[1] persuasion is a therapeutic process in which certain effects are produced by chains of logical reasoning, and he distinguishes it sharply from suggestion. He does not deny the potency of the latter, but believes it to be capable only of evil, and he ascribes to it most of the symptoms occurring in the neuropathic conditions which he treats. Persuasion, on the other hand, does not trade upon the blind credulity of the patient, but enables him to understand the erroneous lines along which his thoughts have proceeded, and the way in which suggestions have produced an appearance of illness which is not really there; and it thereby gives him the necessary means to correct these morbid effects. Dubois' conception is almost entirely intellectualistic, and ascribes to reason a power as a driving force which it very certainly does not possess. It is an unquestionable fact that his method achieves results, but we are compelled to believe that this is because driving forces other than reason are interpolated, of which the suggestive potency of the physician's personality is probably the most frequent and important.

[1] Dubois, *The Psychic Treatment of Nervous Disorders*, English translation, 1909.

In so far, however, as this suggestive action calls to its aid the patient's understanding, instead of merely dumping into his mind a belief without connexions or logical supports, persuasion may be said to be more integrative than simple suggestion, and to this extent superior to it.

Dejerine[1] is less intellectualistic than Dubois, and appreciates the weakness of reason as a driving force. His conception of persuasion includes not only the logical processes of Dubois, but also the principle that an "emotion" must be introduced in order to make these logical processes effective. He repudiates suggestion as a producer of evil almost as energetically as Dubois, but it is difficult to see how his conception of an emotional persuasion differs in its essentials from that of suggestion. His book is full of useful practical details of treatment, but his etiological theories are not very precise. He ascribes a number of conditions to what he terms "preoccupation," citing, for example, the frequent functional disturbances of digestive and other organs which may arise from the patient becoming "preoccupied with," i.e. having his attention fixed upon, the organ in question; and the consequent development of fears and apprehensions, which ultimately produce the neurosis. There can be no question that this conception of Dejerine's does apply to many cases, and that its application points the way to some valuable psychotherapeutic procedures. If we examine the conception itself, however, it does not seem to be materially different from that of suggestion, and adds but little to the limited understanding of our cases which suggestion is already able to offer. We may indeed sum up the whole contribution to psychopathology of the persuasionist schools as an elaboration of the suggestionist theories, except in so far as these schools have to some extent become permeated by more basic conceptions taken over from other investigators, whose

[1] Dejerine and Gauckler, *The Psychoneuroses and their Treatment by Psychotherapy*, English translation, 1913.

methods of attack have been altogether distinct. It is the work of these other investigators which has been chiefly responsible for the building of modern psychopathology, and to understand that building we must go back to the last decade of the nineteenth century, and trace out the lines of development which diverged from the simple study of suggestion after the time of Charcot, in particular the dissociation conception of Janet, and the dynamic conception of Freud.

The immensely important contribution of Janet may be said to have arisen from the blending of two fields of inquiry, the study of hypnotism on the one hand, and that of hysteria on the other hand, both of which had come within the purview of Janet's teacher, Charcot. We have already dealt with the development of hypnotism, but something must now be said of the history of hysteria, and the views of that disorder which held the field at the time when Janet commenced his investigations.

In ancient medicine the phenomena of hysteria were explained by that demonological conception under which all pictures of disease were subsumed, but this magicoreligious view seems to have clung longer to hysteria than to other disorders. Its influence was rampant in the middle ages, when many hysterical symptoms were regarded as the characteristics of witchcraft, and others were believed to be the result of possession by benign or malignant spirits. The first divergence from the demonological conception, however, is to be found in what may be called the metaphysiological speculations of the Greeks. For Hippocrates hysteria was due to the wanderings of the uterus about the body in search of humidity, and the pressures thereby exerted upon other organs explained the various symptoms observed. Coma and lethargy, for example, arose from pressure on the vessels mounting to the head, suffocation from pressure on the bronchial tubes, palpitations from pressure on the heart, and epigastric oppression from pressure on the liver. Galen rejected the Hippocratic theory on the very solid ground that the anatomical fixations of the uterus did not permit of its wandering about the body, but he substituted for it the scarcely better founded view that hysteria was the result of engorgement of the uterus by its own fluid or by menstrual blood. Except for the demonological interlude of the middle ages this uterine pathology persisted in various guises down to the seventeenth century, when Lepois[1] in France and Thomas Willis[2] in this country first put forward the conception that the seat of hysteria was in the brain. The views of Willis are of interest to us here because he observed the causal relationship existing between emotional disturbances and hysteria, but he held that the former acted upon the brain by way of the "animal spirits" which, with the other writers of his time, he regarded as the moving force of nervous action, and therefore his view is essentially physiological and not psychological. Sydenham[3] held that hysteria was a general malady of the nervous system, but here again he supposed this to consist in a disorder of the part producing "animal spirits."

The history of hysteria before Charcot may be said to have culminated in the work of Briquet, who, in his *Traité de l'Hystérie*, published in 1859, reviewed all the theories which had hitherto been put forward, and tested them in the light of his own observations. Briquet's methods were admirably conceived, and they constitute perhaps the first clear attempt to apply to this sphere the rigid procedure of science. He constantly emphasises the importance of unbiassed observations of facts and the avoidance of *a priori* theories, and strives to base his own views entirely on the careful examination of his 430 cases. He finally concludes that "hysteria is a malady consisting in a neurosis of the portion of the brain

---

[1] Lepois, *Morbus qui vulgo dicitur hysteria*, 1620.
[2] Willis, *Opera medica: Pathologia cerebri et nervosi generis*, 1660.
[3] Sydenham, *Dissertatio epistolaris ad B. Coole*.

destined to receive the affective impressions and the sensations."[1] It will be noted that, although this definition contains some psychological terms, it is essentially conceived in a physiological spirit, and is pathological rather than psychopathological. This view may be said, indeed, to have persisted as the doctrine of "functional nervous disorder" which held the field until comparatively recent times.

Charcot noted that in certain cases of traumatic hysteria the physical accident was not in itself the cause of the illness, but that a part was played by the memories left by the accident, and finally he proposed the view that certain of the symptoms of hysteria were due to "ideas." With this view was laid the foundation stone of the psychopathological conception of hysteria, and here also we see the beginning of a delimitation of "psychogenic" from other diseases. Charcot himself, however, did not follow out his observation to its logical consequences, but strove constantly to bring hysteria into line with organic nervous disorder. He related its phenomena to those of hypnosis, and observed the effect of suggestion in both, but he regarded hysteria as a definite disease characterised by definite stigmata. He arrived, indeed, at a conception which was the converse of the later one of Babinski, in that he held hypnosis to be a manifestation of hysteria, and therefore to be part of a disease in which suggestibility appeared, but did not constitute its essence.

Nevertheless the seed which Charcot had sown fell upon fertile ground, and was developed into a rich harvest by the researches of Janet[2]. He found that the

---

[1] Briquet, *Traité clinique et thérapeutique de l'hystérie*, 1859, p. 601: "...l'hystérie est une maladie consistant dans une névrose de la portion d'encéphale destinée à recevoir les impressions affectives et les sensations."

[2] Janet's chief works are *L'Automatisme psychologique*, 1889; *État mental des hystériques*, 1892, English translation *The mental state of hystericals*, 1901; *Névroses et idées fixes*, 1897; *Les Obsessions et la Psychasthénie*, 1903; *Les médications psychologiques*, 1919, translation *Psychological Healing*, 1925.

phenomena of hysteria were capable of being interpreted
in psychological terms, and he finally succeeded in formu-
lating psychopathological conceptions which served, at
any rate in some measure, to explain those phenomena.
The nature and importance of these conceptions will be
best understood if a brief description is given of Janet's
observations and conclusions with regard to a single
group of hysterical symptoms, and for this purpose the
familiar anaesthesias may be selected.

In the first place, Janet noted that hysterical anaesthesia frequently had a peculiar distribution. The well-
known glove anaesthesia, for example, ending in a sharp
line at the level of the wrist, had a distribution which
did not correspond to any possible lesion of the nervous
system, but which did correspond precisely to something,
namely the patient's idea of his own hand. Clearly,
therefore, the incidence of this symptom was determined
by a factor of a psychological order and, if this were so,
it would be profitable to seek for a psychological conception in order to explain it. Again, these anaesthesias
exhibited features of a curiously paradoxical character.
It was observed that patients suffering from extensive
hysterical anaesthesias involving large areas of the body
rarely sustained any accidental injury, whereas patients
with far smaller anaesthesias of organic origin, such as
occur for example in syringo-myelia, frequently sustained
such injury. The only conclusion possible would seem
to be that the patients must feel with their anaesthetic
limbs, as otherwise injury would inevitably befall them.
Similarly, it was found that patients with an extreme
hysterical amblyopia which reduced the field of vision
almost to a single point, were able to play at ball, a performance obviously out of the question unless the major
part of the retina were functioning normally. This paradoxical character appeared most clearly, perhaps, in the
case of a boy who developed hysterical symptoms after
being concerned in a fire. The symptoms were of two

kinds, firstly the presence of an amblyopia which cut down the field of vision in both eyes to 30°, secondly the occurrence of fits, which were originated whenever the patient saw a burning object. Now if the boy were tested with a perimeter in the usual way he was unable to see the paper disc until it had reached the 30° radius. Nevertheless, if a lighted match were substituted for the paper disc, a fit invariably occurred as soon as the match reached the limit of normal vision. Obviously, therefore, the patient could see over the whole field of vision, and equally obviously he was blind to everything outside 30°.

In order to explain these features Janet devised the conception of "dissociation of consciousness." He assumed that consciousness, instead of pursuing its course as a unitary stream could be split into two or more independent currents, so that the consciousness of one current would be unaware of, and uncontrollable by, the consciousness of other contemporaneous currents. Some approximation to this situation occurs normally when we carry out at the same time two independent activities, such as playing the piano and thinking out some problem, but in hysteria the dissociation may reach an extreme degree. Here the sensations arising from an entire limb may be diverted into a current separated from the main stream of consciousness, thereby producing an anaesthesia. Although thus cut off, and incapable of being perceived by the main stream, they can influence the motor apparatus, and thereby determine the phenomena observed, the avoidance of injury by the anaesthetic patient, and the fits in the blind boy. In this way the apparent paradox, that the sensations exist and yet do not exist, can be resolved. The conception of dissociation therefore explains the observed facts, but if it is to satisfy the canons of scientific method, it must also be capable of verification by an appeal to experience. Actually it does satisfy this further test because, if a method be devised whereby access to the dissociated portion can be obtained, the continued existence of the apparently absent sensations can be experimentally demonstrated. By using the manœuvre known as automatic writing, for example, the anaesthetic arm can be made to record, unknown to the patient, the fact that it is being pricked.

Functional paralyses are similarly explicable, as is also hysterical amnesia. The latter consists in a loss of memory for a certain defined period of the patient's life, extending over days, months, or years, and was a common phenomenon in the psychoneuroses of the War. Here again the conception of dissociation presumes that the missing memories are not destroyed, but diverted into a current split off from the main stream of consciousness, and once more the validity of this conception can be experimentally demonstrated by hypnotising the patient, and thus recovering the lost memories.

Other hysterical phenomena, such as somnambulisms and double personalities, can be explained by a dissociation essentially identical with that responsible for amnesias, but differing in its mode of incidence. In these cases a dissociated current suddenly usurps the field of consciousness, causing a complete break in the continuity of the patient's experience and behaviour. After occupying the stage for a certain period of time the dissociated current is once more submerged, and the patient resumes the thread of his former life, generally without any awareness that it has been interrupted. Hysterical somnambulisms can be closely paralleled by certain conditions artificially produced under hypnosis, and a number of the processes occurring in hypnosis, particularly in its more profound phases, are to be interpreted in terms of dissociation.

The conception of dissociation cast a flood of light on a mass of phenomena which had hitherto baffled all attempts at explanation. It was legitimately constructed according to the canons of science by the careful collection of observed facts, and the devising of a formula which would resume those facts. It could, moreover, be tested to any desired extent by constantly comparing the results capable of being deduced from the formula with those actually found by experience and experiment. Finally it pointed out a road along which therapeutic attempts might hopefully be prosecuted. Certain difficulties have been noted in the application of the concept to some of the phenomena with which it is concerned, but these are due rather to misapprehension of the nature of the concept than to defects in the concept itself. For example, in many cases of hypnotic somnambulism the hypnotic consciousness is aware of the whole range of the patient's experience, whereas what we may call the normal consciousness has no knowledge of the experience belonging to the hypnotic consciousness. At first sight this one-sided and non-reciprocal lack of awareness may seem difficult to explain by dissociation, which would appear necessarily to involve a break between the two streams of consciousness equally untraversable in whichever direction it might be attempted, whereas in the example cited the break is impassable when viewed from the side of the normal consciousness, but traversable with ease when viewed from the side of the hypnotic consciousness. The difficulty is dependent, however, upon a misconception of the nature of dissociation, and an abuse of the spatial metaphor in which it is defined. Dissociation does not, of course, imply an actual separation in space, and from the nature of the phenomena with which it is concerned it obviously can have no real spatial significance whatever. Spatial terms are used because they afford a useful method of describing relationship, but actually the dissociation is a functional dissociation, an "out of gear" relationship, and if this is understood the existence of a non-reciprocal dissociation ceases to be inexplicable[1].

Janet's conception of dissociation involves necessarily another conception concerning which something must be

[1] Cf. pp. 162–163.

said, that of the "subconscious." This term has been used in a variety of senses by different authors, but in Janet's work it indicates the existence, contemporaneously with the main stream of consciousness, of mental processes which are independent of and unconnected with the main stream. In this sense it will be apparent that subconsciousness is merely a corollary of dissociation, for a mental process which exists independently of the main stream of consciousness is a dissociated mental process. The conception of the subconscious has been attacked on the ground that processes which are not part of the personal consciousness are not conscious at all, that they are merely neurological or physiological, and have no psychological aspect. This criticism arises from a complete misunderstanding of the nature and justification of a psychological conception. In the first place the evidence for the existence of Janet's subconscious processes is precisely the same as the evidence for the existence of any conscious processes whatever. Both are dependent upon inferences from observed facts. If I see my neighbour writing certain words I infer the existence in him of certain conscious processes, but I have no direct experience of the latter; the only objective facts are the words and the actions I see. Similarly if, as occurs in "automatic writing," a patient's arm writes a coherent and relevant statement, although the patient himself has no knowledge of the fact that his arm is so engaged, or of the subject upon which it writes, I have as much right to attribute consciousness to the mechanism responsible for the statement written by the arm, as I have to attribute consciousness to any other aspect of the patient's behaviour[1]. Secondly the observed facts are not in

[1] It must of course be noted that Janet's conception of the subconscious is to be sharply distinguished from the conception of the "unconscious," and that the foregoing argument is not applicable to the latter. The "unconscious" will be discussed subsequently. A more detailed treatment of both these conceptions, and of their relationship, will be found in the author's "The

themselves either physiological or psychological; they are behaviour facts, and the physiological or psychological aspect is only introduced when an attempt is made to devise conceptions to explain them. If explanation is attempted in terms of nerve cells and fibres a physiological conception is employed, if in terms of ideas and memories a psychological conception is employed. It is not that either conception is wrong: both are permissible, and the choice between them on scientific grounds depends entirely upon their relative utility in enabling us to resume and control the facts of experience. To object, therefore, that the facts which Janet interprets by his conception of the subconscious are physiological and not psychological is irrelevant, and indeed meaningless. The only question at issue is whether, in the present state of our knowledge, a psychological conception such as Janet's permits us to understand, to predict, and to control, the facts of hysteria and hypnotism better than a physiological conception. To this question there can only be one answer, although we are quite entitled to hope that ultimately a physiological explanation still more adequate and useful will be devised.

Morton Prince has explored the field opened up by Janet in several interesting directions, and has applied the concept of dissociation to the study of a wide range of phenomena. He has indeed used the experimental method in psychopathology more consistently than any other investigator, and his work is a valuable object lesson of what can be accomplished by this method. In particular his fascinating *Dissociation of a Personality*[1] provides a convincing demonstration of the light which

conception of the Subconscious," *Journ. of Abnorm. Psychol.* 1909, reprinted in Morton Prince's *Subconscious Phenomena*, 1915. An abstract of the chief conclusions reached in this paper has been incorporated in the appendix on "The conceptions of the subconscious, coconscious, and unconscious" which will be found at the end of the present lecture (see p. 57).

[1] Morton Prince, *The Dissociation of a Personality*, 1906.

the conception of dissociation is able to throw on the problems of double personality, although, as we shall see later, it also affords an excellent example of the limitations of that conception.

Janet has himself extended the conception of dissociation to a wider field than that of hysteria and hypnosis. He brought into a single disease-entity, under the name of "psychasthenia," practically all the manifestations of the psychoneuroses other than the definitely hysterical. In its symptomatology were included phobias, obsessions, compulsive actions of all kinds, morbid anxiety, and states of doubt and hesitation. This remarkable generalisation gathered together a multitude of syndromes which had hitherto been described as independent disorders under such names as "folie de doute," agoraphobia, and so forth, and conceived them all to be merely different aspects of one and the same essential disturbance. The essential disturbance consisted in a dissociation analogous to that responsible for hysteria, although differing from the latter in certain important respects. Starting from the assumption that normal adaptation to reality requires the integration of a number of relevant mental processes, Janet held that both hysteria and psychasthenia are due to a failure of this necessary integration owing to the presence of dissociation. In the case of hysteria the dissociation is molar, that is to say masses of processes are entirely split off from the main stream, thus producing the anaesthesias, paralyses, and somnambulisms. In the case of psychasthenia, on the other hand, the dissociation is molecular, the various processes not being completely segregated from one another, but merely loosened in their interconnexions, so that the firm integration required for efficient adaptation to reality cannot be obtained. In Janet's *Les Obsessions et la Psychasthénie* this principle is worked out in an extraordinarily ingenious manner, and it cannot be denied that it has some value as an explanatory concept. Nevertheless, although it gives us a measure of help and understanding in this complex and difficult field, there is little doubt that the conception of molecular dissociation is unduly wide, and describes a process so elementary and universal that it brings together diverse clinical pictures between which only a superficial resemblance can be traced. We see here, as we have already seen in the case of suggestion, that besetting tendency to generalise a valuable conception until its explanatory value becomes seriously impaired.

We may now pause to consider the place in psychopathology of the conception of dissociation. Even in the wide sense which has just been discussed it has a certain value in that it emphasises the important principle that the processes composing mental activity are not uniformly bound together into a single stream, but may possess varying degrees of independence, a principle which gives us some understanding, not only of psychasthenia, but also of the hallucinations, delusions, and other phenomena met with in the psychoses. It has been said, however, that this principle is so general in its application that it does not give much help in the interpretation of individual pictures of disease, and dissociation will therefore be a more valuable concept if it is limited to the original sense in which Janet brought it forward to explain the symptoms of hysteria. There is no necessity to recapitulate the merits of this conception, and the light that it has shed on the understanding and control of certain phenomena. Something must be said, however, concerning its limitations and defects. To begin with, it does not seem to be applicable to all the phenomena which occur in hysteria. It explains the anaesthesias, for example, but hardly the hyperaesthesias. On the other hand, it explains conditions which occur outside the range of hysteria, such as the automatisms of epilepsy. Janet may be said, indeed, to have discovered a concept of considerable value throughout the whole range of psychopathology, rather than one which will explain all the phenomena of any one part thereof. Secondly, its explanatory value is limited. It enables us to understand that the characters of hysterical anaesthesia or paralysis are due to a splitting of consciousness, but we are immediately faced with the further problem as to *why* this splitting takes place. Dissociation may in fact be regarded as an "anatomical" as opposed to a "functional" conception. This is well seen in Prince's *Dissociation of a Personality*. In it we have an illuminating analysis whereby the speech and behaviour of a patient is shown to be a manifestation of the activities of a number of distinct personalities, but the question as to the conditions responsible for this splitting, in other words, why the dissociation has occurred, is left without satisfactory answer. Dissociation therefore takes us a certain distance in the understanding of our patients, but leaves us with the further problem of explaining the dissociation itself[1].

Janet has himself appreciated this limitation, and sought to overcome it by his doctrine of "psychological tension." This is a property which varies in a manner analogous to the pressure of the atmosphere, the variations being produced by constitutional, emotional and other causes. When it is high, mental processes are integrated with comparative ease, and efficient adaptation to reality is attained. When it is low, the required integration is impossible, and dissociation of some kind occurs, either the molar dissociation of hysteria, or the molecular dissociation of psychasthenia. This is not a very satisfying explanation, however, and seems to come perilously near explaining the incidence of dissociation by a hypothetical faculty of dissociability. It is true that Janet has gone further in that he has emphasised the part played by emotions and the automatic development of affectively toned "idées fixes,"

[1] A further consideration of the conception of dissociation and its relation to the later concepts of Freud will be found in the author's paper on "The Conception of Dissociation" which has been reprinted as the final chapter of the present volume (pp. 154–175).

and may be said therefore to be the forerunner of the dynamic interpretation of the psychoneuroses, but this dynamic aspect is not clearly followed up.

The stage in the history of psychopathology marked by the conception of dissociation is comparable to that existing in the history of astronomy at the time of Kepler. Kepler had shown that the planets move in ellipses round the sun, but he could not explain why they did so. This latter achievement was the work of Newton with his formulation of the law of gravity. Newton's step was based on the conception that the phenomena observed were the result of certain hypothetical forces, interacting in accordance with certain precisely definable laws. It thus added a dynamic conception as a means of understanding the observed sequence of phenomena. The corresponding step in the construction of a psychological conception capable of taking us beyond the level reached by dissociation, clearly required a similar advance to a dynamic point of view, and it is the attempt to make this advance which actually characterises the later history of psychopathology.

The dynamic conception in psychopathology has derived its chief impetus from the work of Freud, but it must not be forgotten that a parallel dynamic aspect made its appearance in academic psychology with the development of the conception of instinct. The view that instinct, or rather various instincts, can be regarded as driving forces whose action and interaction produce the mental phenomena and behaviour of man, has received its best-known expression in the work of McDougall. He defines instinct as "an inherited or innate psychophysical disposition which determines its possessor to perceive, and to pay attention to, objects of a certain class, to experience an emotional excitement of a particular quality upon perceiving such an object, and to act in regard to it in a particular manner, or, at least, to experience an impulse to such action,"[1] For example,

[1] McDougall, *An Introduction to Social Psychology*, 16th edition, 1921, p. 29.

the instinct of flight determines us to perceive dangerous objects or situations, to experience the emotion of fear, and to act in a manner which will remove us from the source of danger. This definition is open to criticism, and especially is it doubtful whether the position assigned therein to emotion is correct. It would seem that emotion is manifested when the action of an instinct is inhibited, e.g. fear when it is not possible to remove ourselves from the source of danger, rather than in the normal course of an unobstructed instinct. We are not concerned here with details of this character, however, but only with the general conception of instinct as a driving force capable of explaining the activity of man. It is clear that psychology has thus obtained a dynamic conception enabling it to emerge from the arid paths of academic introspection and mere description to which it was so long condemned. By the aid of this dynamic standpoint a vista is opened up whereby psychology is no longer limited to recording the "how" of the phenomena with which it deals, but can attempt an answer to the question "Why?" It can attempt to conceive the sequence of thought and behaviour in man as a result of the interplay of various instinctive forces acting according to precisely definable laws, and if this attempt is successful psychology will have been lifted from the level of a descriptive science to that long ago attained by such sciences as chemistry and physics.

The question immediately arises, however, whether a psychological conception of this character is permissible in science. The naïve notion that it deals with flimsy abstractions unworthy of being ranked with such solid realities as electrons and ether waves has already been discussed, but there is a more substantial difficulty to be considered. The conception has a teleological aspect, and introduces an element which is not only psychological but which has no correlate or parallel in physics, namely, the element of "purpose." According to McDougall an instinctive process is not completely explained by a *vis a tergo*. It not only moves towards an end, but the existence of that end is a determining factor throughout, and may continually modify the process during its whole course. In other words the process not merely happens to serve a purpose, but is actually in part determined by that purpose. Now it is sometimes held that the introduction of purpose as a determining factor is incompatible with the notion of causality, and that, as causality is the foundation stone of scientific method, no conception involving purpose can have a place in science[1]. A long war has been waged against this mechanistic limitation of science and, although it is obviously impossible here to deal with the subject adequately, something must be said, because to admit this limitation would necessitate the expulsion of modern psychopathology from the domain of science.

Psychological conceptions are characterised by the fact that they are couched in terms of experience and, as purpose is clearly an integral part of our experience, there is no objection on this score to the incorporation of purpose in a psychological conception. The further question whether purpose is consonant or incompatible with causality requires for its answer a precise definition of this latter word, and it is apparent that it is used in two senses which are by no means identical[2]. In one sense it indicates an unconditional sequence, the fact that *a* is inevitably followed by *b*. In this sense there seems to be no reason why purpose should be excluded from causality; it takes its place as one of the factors determining a particular sequence of phenomena. If we can ascertain the existence of this and the other conditioning

---

[1] This is the standpoint taken by Jung. Cf. Jung, *Analytical Psychology*, 2nd edition, 1917, pp. x and xv. A vindication of "purpose" as an integral factor in psychology will be found in McDougall, *An Outline of Psychology*, 1923.

[2] Höffding, *The Problems of Philosophy*, 1905, p. 66.

factors, and are acquainted with their laws of action, we can predict the course of future phenomena, and thus satisfy the essential criterion of the method of science. There is a second sense, however, in which the word causality is used. Here it indicates not merely inevitable succession, but a relation of identity between cause and effect. The effect is regarded as the cause in a new form. For example, when we say that heat is the cause of motion, we mean that motion is the equivalent of heat in a new form. Heat is conceived as being the vibration of particles, and hence motion can be regarded as a continuation of the same phenomenon. In this sense causality is an equation, and one which is essentially reversible, so that the sequence of cause and effect can be equally well replaced by the sequence of effect and cause. This is the sense in which causality is understood in the mechanistic sciences, and it would seem that it cannot be applied to purposive psychology, for a sequence in which purpose is playing a part is clearly not reversible, and cannot be regarded as an equation. The introduction of purpose, therefore, removes psychology from the mechanistic sciences, but this does not justify its removal from the whole field of science. The method of science requires the assumption of causality in the first sense, but not necessarily in the second sense, and in the first sense causality is as integral a part of purposive psychology as it is of any other branch of science. If it were insisted that causality in the second sense is an essential constituent of science, then not only psychology, but physiology and biology also, would have to be excluded, because in the conceptions of all branches of knowledge dealing with life processes irreversibility of the sequences has necessarily to be admitted. The inapplicability of the narrower concept of causality is not therefore a peculiarity of psychology, but a peculiarity of all the biological sciences, and the circumstances we have considered merely indicate that psychology is extra-mechanistic, but not extra-scientific.

This digression has been necessary in order to justify the incorporation into science of conceptions involving the element of purpose, and we may now return to the later history of psychopathology in which conceptions of this character play a prominent part. This later history is inseparably bound up with the work of Freud, to whom the most noteworthy advances in psychopathology are unquestionably due, whatever view we may ultimately reach concerning the validity of many of his doctrines.

Freud's conceptions have undergone an extensive development during the course of his career, and it is impossible here either to trace out this development in detail, or to give any adequate account of his theories as they stand to-day. An acquaintance with their general characters must be assumed, and we shall select for consideration only certain broad features which are relevant to our present problem[1].

In 1880 Josef Breuer of Vienna investigated a case of hysteria in which he observed the traumatic effect of certain memories of which the patient was unconscious, and the therapeutic result obtained by bringing these memories once more into consciousness. This investigation, although it was not published until many years later, was the starting point of Freud's work. In 1893 he brought out in association with Breuer a preliminary paper, and in 1895 the *Studien über Hysterie*, which may be said to express the first stage of Freud's development. The keynote of this stage, the view that "the hysteric suffers mainly from reminiscences," is not essentially

[1] Freud's chief works are *Studien über Hysterie* (with Breuer), 1895; *Die Traumdeutung*, 1900; *Zur Psychopathologie des Alltagslebens*, 1901; *Drei Abhandlungen zur Sexualtheorie*, 1905; numerous shorter papers collected into five *Sammlungen kleiner Schriften zur Neurosenlehre*; *Vorlesungen zur Einführung in die Psychoanalyse*, 1917; *Jenseits des Lustprinzips*, 1920; *Massenpsychologie und Ich-Analyse*, 1921; *Das Ich und das Es*, 1923. Practically all have now been translated into English.

different from Janet's notion of "idées fixes," which certainly preceded in time Breuer and Freud's publication, although it is claimed that the latter had a quite independent origin. There is apparent in the work of Breuer and Freud, however, a much more definite dynamic formulation than Janet had attained, and new conceptions of fundamental importance, such as "repression" and "resistance," were laid down. To this period belongs the use of hypnosis as a method of recovering buried memories, the conception of "psychic trauma," and treatment by "catharsis," that is to say, the bringing to consciousness of the traumatic memory and its "abreaction" by allowing it to obtain the normal emotional expression which had formerly been denied to it. We need not concern ourselves here with these conceptions, except to note that hypnosis was abandoned by Freud many years ago, as was also the notion of "psychic trauma," and that treatment by catharsis only bears a remote resemblance to the modern method of psychoanalysis.

After the dissolution of the partnership between Breuer and Freud the latter proceeded independently, and produced a succession of works in which the earlier conceptions were considerably modified, extended, and made more systematic and precise. Although the development has been continuous it will be convenient to postpone for the moment the consideration of the later additions, and to devote our attention to the theories as they stood before the War. The essential structure, with which we are alone concerned, remains the same to-day, but it is easier to see and to examine without the accretions and amplifications of the last decade.

This essential structure may be very briefly and inadequately sketched as follows. The phenomena of conscious life and behaviour are conceived as the result of the interaction of a number of psychological "forces," which interact according to precisely definable "laws." These forces, which are in part conscious and in part unconscious, may work harmoniously together, or they may conflict with one another. In the latter case an attempt at adjustment occurs, and this attempt may proceed in various possible ways. Certain of these ways involve the repression of one of the opposing forces, that is to say one of the forces is put out of gear, as it were, and is no longer allowed to manifest itself normally in consciousness or in action. It becomes unconscious, but does not thereby cease to exist or to be capable of functioning. It can no longer influence thought and behaviour in a normally direct manner, but it produces various indirect effects. For example, the sex instincts in an elderly unmarried woman, repressed because of their incompatibility with her moral code, and with the circumstances of her life, may express themselves in consciousness as an abnormal interest in births, marriages, and scandals. These indirect effects manifest themselves by means of certain mechanisms which Freud precisely defines, such as compromise, condensation, representation by the opposite, and so forth. Mechanisms of this character are responsible for many phenomena in everyday life, slips of the pen and of speech for instance, for the content of dreams, and for the various symptoms manifested in the psychoneuroses.

It must be understood that the foregoing is only an attempt to describe in general terms the supporting columns on which Freud's theories appear to rest, and does not correspond to the actual way in which these theories were developed. Freud's attack was purely empirical, and he subjected the psychoneuroses to a prolonged clinical study, only slowly and tentatively building up theoretical conceptions to account for the phenomena which he had observed. It will be noted that, in form at least, this course is entirely irreproachable from the standpoint of the canons of science. After his abandonment of hypnotism as a means of investigation he evolved the method of psychoanalysis, and it is by the use of this method that practically all the facts of observation upon which the Freudian theories rest have been collected. We shall have subsequently to describe it, and to evaluate its claim to rank as a trustworthy instrument of research. At present, however, we are concerned with the results of its employment, rather than with the instrument itself.

In the course of his psychoanalytic investigations of the phenomena of the psychoneuroses Freud noted that the conflicts underlying the symptoms were invariably conflicts between forces belonging to two radically distinct groups. The first group comprised forces apparently emanating from the sex instincts, the second group forces connected with the personality. To the first Freud gave the name of "libido," to the second that of "the ego," and he conceived that a psychoneurosis developed owing to a certain failure of adjustment between these two or, as he has himself expressed it, "when the Ego loses its capacity to deal in some way or other with the Libido."[1] In view of the important part played by the libido Freud subjected this to a careful examination in order to determine its precise mode of development, and as a result of this examination he reached the remarkable conclusions constituting the well-known " sexual theories." According to these theories sex as we know it in the adult is not a function which suddenly emerges at puberty in a manner comparable to the birth of Minerva, but is the final stage in a long process of development starting from the dawn of life. Although its early manifestations are very different from the adult function the term sexual can justly be applied to the former, because the latter is clearly developed therefrom. Moreover many tendencies not generally regarded as sexual, for example parental and filial love, and indeed all the processes to which the word "love" can be applied, must similarly be brought

[1] Freud, *Introductory Lectures on Psychoanalysis*, English translation, 1922, p. 323.

within the sphere of the libido, because they also can be shown to originate from the common fount. The earlier stages in the development of the libido are distinguished by differences both in the objects towards which the libido is directed, and in the parts of the body with which the libido is associated, and these differences characterise definite stages through which the libido passes in its progress to adult normality. Thus in the earliest stages the libido is directed on to the individual himself, later on to one or both parents, and only in its final development is it directed on to other persons of the opposite sex. Similarly in earlier stages the libido is associated with parts of the body other than the genitalia, for example the mouth and anus, and only later does the genital zone assume the primacy which characterises adult sex.

Freud observed that the psychoneuroses were associated with a failure in this process of development, the normal evolution being partially arrested at an early stage. A very important stage in this respect was that at which the libido was directed on to one of the parents, generally the parent of the opposite sex. A failure of adequate development here meant that the libido was fixated at this stage, and could not undergo its normal evolution. This fixation was invariably found in certain types of psychoneurosis, and the conflict, which resulted when the claims of later life demanded a normal distribution of the libido, was responsible for the outbreak of the symptoms. In other conditions fixations at other levels were found to be present, and in a word the whole structure and development of the psychoneuroses could be worked out in each individual case by the application of these conceptions.

This description, condensed and generalised to an extent which is hardly consistent with accuracy, will have to serve for our immediate purpose, namely the estimation of the Freudian theories, both in their form and content, by the canons of scientific method. To begin with, it is clear that with conceptions of this character a goal has been aimed at far beyond that achieved by the dissociation conception of Janet. The essential mark of the advance lies in the move forward to a dynamic point of view, and the endeavour to account for the observed phenomena by the action of precise forces working according to precisely definable laws. Similarly the goal attempted is far beyond that reached by the suggestionist and persuasionist schools because, although suggestion is a dynamic concept, it is immeasurably inferior in precision and manageability to the concepts which Freud has constructed. It is unnecessary to point out, therefore, that Freud's attempt is a very notable one, and if it can be established either in whole or in part, it must rank amongst the great achievements of the world. The importance of ascertaining how far his methods are consonant with the method of science, and how far the observed facts justify his conclusions, cannot be overestimated, and the magnitude of the issue requires that this should be done with the utmost care and consideration. We may endeavour to approach the problem by a preliminary examination of certain of Freud's fundamental conceptions, and may take in order the conception of the unconscious, the mechanisms, and the sex theories.

The conception of the unconscious is an integral part of Freud's theories. He holds that the processes we term conscious are only a superficial layer, as it were, of the total sum of mental processes. There are two other layers, the pre-conscious, comprising those processes which although not conscious at the moment may at any time become so, and the unconscious, comprising processes which are not only not conscious at the moment, but are prevented from becoming conscious by a barrier only to be circumvented under special circumstances. The unconscious processes are nevertheless able to influence consciousness in various indirect ways. Freud formulates very precisely the nature, characters, and mode of action of the processes contained in the unconscious.

The conception of the unconscious has been subjected to much adverse criticism. It is said that it involves a contradiction in terms, as consciousness is the essential character of mental processes, and an unconscious mental process therefore an absurdity; that the processes in question are not psychological at all, but physiological, and that they should be conceived not in terms of consciousness, but in terms of brain. These criticisms arise from a confusion of thought. The unconscious is not a phenomenal reality, but a concept fashioned in order to explain the phenomenal reality. The phenomenal reality, consciousness, obviously forms a disconnected series and, if the psychologist is compelled to take only this into account, he cannot rise beyond the level of a mere description of psychic phenomena. To obtain understanding and continuity it is necessary to go beyond the phenomena and to construct an explanatory concept. The physiologist has of course a perfect right to construct for this purpose a concept in terms of brain, but he cannot deny to the psychologist an equal right to construct a concept in psychological terms. The question is not whether one is correct and the other incorrect, but which one works the best in the present state of our knowledge. So far as the phenomena which Freud seeks to explain are concerned the physiologist cannot yet give an explanation which consists of more than words, and the fact that these words indicate hypothetical material processes rather than hypothetical psychical processes is an inadequate consolation for his entire inability to make any use of the conceptions he fashions. The psychologist is therefore perfectly justified in attempting to find an explanation by the construction of a psychological conception, at any rate until the physiologist can provide one which is practically more useful, and such a conception must involve the assumption of an unconscious in

one form or another. If consciousness is defined as the
essential attribute of mental processes, then of course
the unconscious becomes a contradiction in terms, but
as the question is already begged by accepting the definition this is not of much moment. We saw, when discussing
Janet's conception of the subconscious, that there is
convincing proof that mental processes exist which are
not personally conscious, and such processes are unconscious from the standpoint of the personal consciousness.
It may be added that, even if the notion of the unconscious were contradicted by our experience of phenomenal
reality this would not necessarily preclude it from ranking
as a scientific concept, because a concept is a constructed
and not a phenomenal entity[1]. An unconscious mental
process, for example, would not be more absurd than a
weightless and frictionless ether. Criticisms directed
against the unconscious as a possible conception do not
carry much weight, therefore, and we have seen that a
conception of this kind is necessary if the psychologist is
to be allowed to explain the phenomena of consciousness
in psychological terms[2]. The question whether Freud's
particular conception of the unconscious is valid is of
course another matter. On the score of method there is
no objection whatever to its form and structure, but to
satisfy the canons of science it must be shown that it is
based on accurately observed facts, that it explains those
facts, and that the deductions which follow from it when
tested by experience and experiment are always found
to be verified. These are the only criteria which have
any relevance if the value of Freud's concept is to be
satisfactorily estimated.

[1] Cf. Lecture I, p. 4.
[2] Freud's conception of the unconscious differs fundamentally
from Janet's "subconscious," and the considerations which justify
the one are not applicable to the other. Cf. p. 39, footnote. See
also the appendix "The conceptions of the subconscious, coconscious, and unconscious," p. 57, in which the nature and relationships of these conceptions are more fully considered.

The mechanisms, that is to say, the modes of action whereby the various intrapsychic forces produce the phenomena they are invoked to explain, need not be considered in detail. Here belong the conceptions of conflict, repression, and the effects upon consciousness and behaviour which a repressed system is capable of producing. This portion of Freud's work has obtained wide acceptance and recognition, extending far beyond the limited circle of Freud's orthodox followers, a circumstance due in some part to the fact that the principles in question were found to be remarkably applicable and illuminating in the study of that great mass of psychoneuroses produced by the War. Here again the conceptions are certainly constructed legitimately so far as their form is concerned, and their validity must be determined, as in the case of the unconscious, by an appeal to the facts and to experience.

In contrast with the comparatively favourable reception accorded to the mechanisms, the sex theories have been the subject of most vigorous attack and rejection. Certain criticisms have been based, sometimes explicitly, but more often implicitly, on ethical or aesthetic grounds. Objections of this kind have, of course, no place or relevancy in positive science, and only require to be mentioned in order that they may be at once dismissed. Other criticisms have more weight. It is held that to reduce all the phenomena of the psychoneuroses to the action of the sex instincts is an unduly narrow view, and that other instinctive forces without admixture of sex elements are equally capable of causing these disorders. It would seem, for example, that the psychoneuroses of the War were certainly due to intrapsychic conflicts, but to conflicts between forces in which sex played no part. We shall see subsequently that the Freudian school has met this latter objection with regard to the war psychoneuroses by a further extension of the already wide denotation ascribed to sex. For the moment, however, it is merely necessary to note that disputes of this kind can only be settled by an appeal to the facts of observation, and not by *a priori* considerations. A generalisation is unduly wide only if it can be shown that the facts do not fit into it, and it is no more inherently impossible that the sex instinct should account for all the phenomena of the psychoneuroses than that so simple a principle as gravity should account for all the movements of the planets. Once more, therefore, we are led to the conclusion that we cannot quarrel with the form in which Freud's sex theories are cast, and that they are legitimate attempts to explain the facts. As in the cases of the unconscious and of the mechanisms, the crux of the matter is whether these conceptions do fit the facts, and fit them in a manner satisfactory to the canons of science. It is unfortunately necessary to labour this simple and obvious point, because many critics of Freud appear to forget that all theories can only be appraised by an examination of the facts, and that, just as a theory can only be legitimately constructed on the careful observation and recording of phenomena, so it can only be destroyed by recapitulating the observations or, as it were, making control experiments. This essential work is often altogether neglected, and its place taken by *ex cathedra* statements, whose foundations in prejudice are sometimes only too obvious. An examination at the level of the facts of observation, therefore, must clearly be the chief task in any reasonable attempt to judge the value of Freud's conceptions.

APPENDIX

THE CONCEPTIONS OF THE SUBCONSCIOUS, COCONSCIOUS, AND UNCONSCIOUS

In the history of psychology the words "subconscious" and "unconscious" have been used in a variety of meanings, and in the hands of different authors they denote concepts which are radically distinct from one another. Owing to this fact the many disputes waged concerning the validity of the concepts in question have frequently been characterised by a remarkable confusion of thought, and it is imperative that these various meanings should be carefully distinguished and collated if we are to arrive at any clear understanding of the aims and achievements of the authors who employ them. An attempt to carry out this task was made by the present writer in a paper entitled "The Conception of the Subconscious," published in the *Journal of Abnormal Psychology* in 1909, and subsequently reprinted in Morton Prince's *Subconscious Phenomena* (Badger, Boston). This appendix is essentially an abstract of the chief conclusions reached therein.

By Stout and others the term "subconscious" is used to denote those marginal portions of the field of consciousness which are not at the moment in the focus of attention, and is practically equivalent to "dimly conscious." "Unconscious" frequently indicates, notably in common parlance, a mere absence of consciousness, such as is applicable for example to sticks and stones or to states of coma occurring in a normally conscious being. These meanings of "subconscious" and "unconscious" have no relation whatever to the special concepts for which the words are now commonly employed in modern psychology and, except for the fact that they are occasionally responsible for an unpardonable confusion in discussion, they would not call for any mention here.

The modern concepts of "subconscious" and "unconscious" are best illustrated by the use of the first in the work of Janet, and of the second in the work of Freud. It cannot be too strongly emphasised that the two concepts are radically distinct, and that they are respectively concerned with entirely different ranges of facts and entirely different methods of approach.

The subconscious of Janet denotes psychical processes

which have all the characters of normal conscious processes except that of integration with the main stream of consciousness, that is to say, it differs from the personally conscious only in the circumstance that it has been subjected to dissociation. It is applied, therefore, to such phenomena as automatic writing, and to the mental processes presumed to be involved in hysterical dissociations such as anaesthesias and amnesias. The existence of subconscious processes is demonstrated by simple observation, and based upon precisely the same grounds as those which satisfy us of the existence of conscious processes in general.

The unconscious of Freud denotes a region of the mind which is assumed to exist behind the façade, as it were, of consciousness. The processes taking place therein have characters essentially different from those possessed by the processes which occur in consciousness, and behave according to essentially different laws. They cannot enter consciousness directly, but they are nevertheless able to influence consciousness, and the processes discernible on the stage of consciousness may be said indeed to be largely a resultant of the interacting forces existing in the unconscious area behind the scenes. These unconscious forces and their interactions cannot be directly observed; their existence, nature, and mode of action are deduced from the phenomena observed in consciousness, and they serve to explain the latter.

The distinction and relationship between Janet's "subconscious" and Freud's "unconscious" will become immediately apparent if consideration is given to their respective positions in the method of science. We have seen that this method comprises three steps[1], the observation and recording of phenomena, the classification of the phenomena observed, and finally the finding of formulae or laws which will serve to resume or "explain" those phenomena. This third step may involve the

[1] Cf. Lecture I, p. 3.

assumption of hypothetical entities which have no demonstrable phenomenal existence. These entities are not observed phenomena but conceptual abstractions, which are constructed in order to explain the observed phenomena, and are valid scientific weapons just because they do fulfil this function. As an example of such hypothetical entities we may cite the ether and its waves.

Now the subconscious of Janet refers to processes which are *phenomenal*, and their existence is established by simple observation. In a demonstration of automatic writing, for example, we converse with a patient whose hand at the same time writes of matters which are unknown to the personal consciousness. We are entitled here to speak of the subconscious phenomena attending the writing just as we speak of the conscious phenomena attending the patient's conversation. Janet himself has remarked, "These diverse acts are identical with those which we are accustomed to observe in persons like ourselves and to explain by the intervention of intelligence. Undoubtedly one may say that a somnambulist is only a mechanical doll, but then we must say the same of every creature. The term 'doubling of consciousness' is not a philosophical explanation; it is a simple clinical observation of a common character which these phenomena present."[1]

The unconscious of Freud is a conception of an altogether different kind. Here we are no longer on the phenomenal plane, we have moved to the conceptual.

[1] Janet, "The Subconscious," *Journ. of Abnorm. Psychol.* June, 1907. It may be maintained that the great majority of the facts of psychology, in that they imply a knowledge of the conscious phenomena of others gained only by inference and not by direct introspective observation, are really conceptual in character. If conceptual is understood in an indefinitely wide sense this is of course true. But such inferred facts are on an altogether different plane to the conceptions of science. Relatively to the latter they are phenomena, just as helium in the sun is a phenomenon. See the further consideration of this peculiarity of the material of psychology in Lecture III, pp. 69 and 70.

Unconscious processes are not phenomenal facts, they are concepts, constructions devised to explain certain phenomena: they have not been found, they have been made. The implicit assumptions underlying Freud's doctrine may be expressed in this way. Certain entities are imagined which may be described as unconscious psychical factors; certain properties are attached to these factors and they are conceived to act and interact according to certain laws. If it is then found that the results deduced from these formulae correspond to the phenomena actually observed in our experience, and that the correspondence is maintained in all the tests and experiments which can be devised, the formulae may be justifiably incorporated into valid scientific theory.

This train of thought is the analogue of that under lying all the great conceptual constructions of physics and chemistry—the atomic theory, and the theory of the ether and its waves. Here, as in these other instances, its validity must be determined by its ability to satisfy the tests of experiment and experience demanded by the method of science. It is clear, however, that these tests are of a totally different character from those required to establish the facts comprised in Janet's description of the subconscious. The latter are phenomena whose occurrence must be recorded by simple observation, the former are not phenomena at all, but conceptual abstractions whose only justification must be that they enable us to resume and to comprehend the phenomena which experience presents to us. Unless this essential distinction is clearly grasped no adequate appraisement of the contributions of Janet and Freud, or of their mutual relationship, is possible, and the failure to appreciate it is responsible for much of the irrelevant criticism which is still frequently to be heard in discussions on these subjects.

The unconscious of Jung stands on the same level as the unconscious of Freud, and is to be regarded as an alternative concept designed to replace the latter. It is again a conceptual abstraction, whose claim to validity must be determined by the methods applicable to all conceptual abstractions.

The "coconscious" of Morton Prince, on the other hand, stands on the same level as Janet's "subconscious," and is indeed largely identical with the latter. Prince considers that the essential character of a coconscious process consists in the fact that it leads an autonomous existence and is not dependent upon the ego. Coconsciousness, therefore, does not necessarily imply that the personal consciousness is unaware of the processes in question. Thus in *The Dissociation of a Personality*[1], one personality knows all the thoughts and actions of a second, but regards them as those of another being. "Coconscious" therefore covers a wider range of phenomena than "subconscious," and this extension provides a valuable bridge to an understanding of the hallucinations and other analogous manifestations observed in certain psychoses[2].

[1] Morton Prince, *The Dissociation of a Personality*, 1906.

[2] The view that the "unconscious" of Freud is a conceptual construction, essentially different in its nature from the phenomenal "subconscious" of Janet, has not been accepted by the Psychoanalytical School. This school maintains that the unconscious is an entity whose phenomenal existence can be maintained on grounds as substantial as those on which the existence of any of the conscious processes of others can be maintained, the evidence in both cases being of a similar inferential character. This contention is considered in the final chapter of the present volume. See pp. 166 ff.

III

In the preceding lecture the basic conceptions underlying Freud's theories were briefly considered, and the
conclusion reached that their scientific validity could
only be determined by an examination of the observed
facts upon which they are based. An attempt must be
made here to indicate the lines along which such an
examination should be directed, but before passing on to
this task it will be advisable to trace Freud's sex-theories
through a further stage in their development, as a better
understanding of the part assigned to sex and libido in
the modern Freudian system will thereby be attained.
This further stage is characterised by the incorporation
of the conception of "narcissism," and its history lies
along two lines of research, the investigation of dementia
praecox and of the psychoneuroses of the War.

The psychoanalytic investigation of dementia praecox
had been to some extent foreshadowed by Freud, but
the first systematic study along these lines was due to
Jung, who in 1907 published his well-known *Psychologie
der Dementia Praecox*. He showed that while many of
the symptoms of dementia praecox closely resembled
those met with in hysteria, and were explicable by almost
identical mechanisms, yet they differed from the latter
in their fixity and immutability. The characteristic
inaccessibility was further investigated in the light of
Freud's libido theory, and was seen to be associated with
an absolute incapacity for "transference," that is to say,
the peculiar affective relationship between physician and
patient upon which all therapy was conceived to depend.
As a result of subsequent work conceptions were devised
by which the inaccessibility of the dementia praecox
patient was brought definitely into relation with the
libido theory, and the theory itself considerably modified
and extended. It was held that the earlier stages of sex

development included a phase in which the libido was directed on to the individual's own "ego." This phase, in which the ego might be said to constitute the "object" of the libido, preceded the phases in which an object was sought in the outer world, and to its manifestations the name of "narcissism" was given. Dementia praecox could then be conceived as involving a regression to the narcissistic stage of sex development, just as the psychoneuroses were regarded as involving regressions to other and later stages of that development. In this way the familiar features of dementia praecox, its curious shut-in character, its divorce from reality, the inaccessibility of the patient, and his tendency to live in a phantasy of his own making, could be explained as direct results of the attachment of the libido to the ego and its consequent imperviousness to the claims of the external world. And in this way also dementia praecox could be subsumed under that interplay of the libido and the ego which has come to be more and more the central point of the Freudian theories.

During the recent War a great mass of illness occurred which, christened at first by the misleading name of "shell shock," came ultimately to be known as the psychoneuroses of war. This change of nomenclature was due to the rapidly won recognition of the psychological origin of these conditions. Indeed it may be said that, whatever else the War has done, it has at least conclusively demonstrated the existence and importance of psychogenic disorder. It was observed that the psychoneuroses of war, although naturally coloured in their symptomatology by the peculiar circumstances of their origin, did not differ in essentials from the psychoneuroses already familiar in civil life. Moreover, investigators noted that the mechanisms which Freud claimed to be responsible for psychoneurotic symptoms were remarkably applicable to the war conditions, and that they were in fact much more obvious and easily demonstrated in the latter, doubtless because of their relatively rapid development and simple character. There seemed to be no doubt that an intrapsychic conflict was at the bottom of the war psychoneuroses, and one which produced its effects according to laws identical with those already described by Freud. Yet the conflicting forces had apparently no relation to sex, but were manifestly concerned with instincts of a totally different character, in particular those ministering to self-preservation. The general effect of these observations was to confirm in a high degree Freud's conceptions of mechanism, while they threw grave doubt upon his generalisation that psychoneuroses invariably involved the sex instincts and were the result of fixations and regressions in the action of the libido. The Freudian school, however, endeavoured to save the position by an application of their new conception of narcissism. The part apparently played in the war psychoneuroses by the instincts of self-preservation was reduced to a manifestation of narcissism, and thus the conflicts which overtly had no relation to sex were brought within the general theory of the libido and its development.

Freud has always insisted, even in his earliest work, that he was attaching to sex a wider significance than that with which it was generally credited. It is clear, however, that in the developments we have just considered, its application has been extended to a far more comprehensive sphere than was contemplated in the original theories. These developments are, indeed, a particular instance of an evolution which characterises the whole of the later growth of the psychoanalytical doctrines. The libido theory has been pushed into further and further fields, and the manifestations of the libido are now held to include, not merely normal sex activity, perverted sex activity, and the psychoneuroses, but a vast mass of human thought and behaviour. Freud's early generalisation that no neuroses can be present with

H

a normal sexual life has been submerged in an immensely wider generalisation which, though not explicitly stated, might be said to run "Without processes having their origin in sexual life the greater part of human activity would cease to exist." As psychoanalytical investigation proceeds, more and more of the behaviour of man is brought under the general conception of the interplay of libido and ego, and it is perhaps not unreasonable to assume that the aim in view is to bring the whole of such behaviour under it. In other words Freud's theories have moved far beyond the department of medicine in which they had their origin. The position now is that the permutations of the libido account for a great number of the phenomena of life, and certain permutations account for some of the phenomena of disease.

We may pause to examine this wide conception, and to consider whether it is inherently possible or justifiable. To begin with it may be noted that, although the attempt to subsume so much of human activity under a single principle naturally arouses immediate criticism, it is not in itself absurd, and is indeed supported by certain general considerations. Drever has remarked that "though perceptual experience is more and more overlaid by the higher mental processes, it always underlies them, and, though control of primitive impulse becomes more and more complex, it is always a control by that which draws its controlling force, ultimately and fundamentally, from primitive impulses, never a control *ab extra*."[1] Pursuing this line of thought it may be said that, if we are to dissect mental processes into constituent parts, and to trace back the driving forces to their elements, the latter must presumably consist of something like the primitive instincts. Similarly, if we accept an evolutionary standpoint, we must build up man's activities from elements to be observed in lower animals, and sex and self-preservation would constitute the chief

[1] Drever, *Instinct in Man*, 2nd edition, 1921, p. 151.

founts from which energy could ultimately be derived. It is therefore not impossible, or even improbable, that a conception will finally be achieved in which the manifold activities of man are reduced to primitive forces, and found to be the result of permutations and combinations amongst those forces. These considerations serve to show that Freud's attempt is at any rate legitimately conceived, but whether it is a successful attempt is of course another matter. We may conclude that here, as in the case of the other conceptions we have examined, *a priori* objections have no weight, and that the whole structure of Freud's work can only be appraised by a careful examination of the facts upon which it is based, and a determination of the extent to which the concepts proposed can be confirmed and verified by those facts.

The application of criticism along such lines is made easier by the circumstance that these are precisely the criteria by which Freud himself is prepared to abide. He has pointed out that "psychoanalytical investigation could not, like a philosophical system, make its appearance with a complete and ready system of doctrine, but had to build up step by step the way to the understanding of psychical complications by the analytic dissection of normal and abnormal phenomena."[1] In other words, the claim is made that psychoanalytical theory is a direct induction from observed facts, and must stand or fall with the accuracy of the facts and the validity of the induction. Such a claim is a legitimate appeal to the bar of science, and justifiable criticism can only concern itself with two questions: (1) are the facts as stated? (2) are the concepts built up thereon valid?

The first question leads us to the kernel of the matter

[1] Freud, *Das Ich und das Es,* 1923, p. 42: "...dass die psychoanalytische Forschung nicht wie ein philosophisches System mit einem vollständigen und fertigen Lehrgebäude auftreten konnte, sondern sich den Weg zum Verständnis der seelischen Komplikationen schrittweise durch die analytische Zergliederung normaler wie abnormer Phänomene bahnen müsste."

at issue, and discloses at once the strength and the weakness of the psychoanalytic position. The contention is put forward that anyone who will investigate a case by Freud's method will find that the facts observed are as Freud states them to be, and it might appear that if this contention could be established the foundations of psychoanalytical theory would be placed beyond dispute. Now there is undoubtedly considerable evidence in support of this statement, though not perhaps that overwhelming evidence which would serve completely to justify it. It may be accepted that the great majority of those who have examined cases by Freud's method have confirmed his observed facts, and this applies even to observers such as Jung, who have drawn from those facts conclusions very different to those of Freud. Yet this acceptance has by no means that complete confirmatory significance which it at first sight appears to carry. We note that the facts are observed by the aid of a particular method, and until we have carefully examined the nature of this method, and its reliability as a weapon of investigation, the value of the facts ascertained by its use cannot be satisfactorily determined, even if it could be shown that all the users of this method have observed identical phenomena.

The method whereby the facts, upon which Freud relies for the building of his theories, are elicited, is the method of psychoanalysis. The patient talks freely about any subject which occurs to him, avoiding so far as possible any deliberate attempt to control or direct the flow of his associations. It is held that these associations are largely conditioned by forces of which the patient is unconscious, and the physician, from his knowledge of mental mechanisms, is enabled to deduce from the material provided by the patient, and the manner of its presentation, the nature and mode of action of the factors responsible for it. These conclusions are utilised by the physician to point out to the patient the significance of certain of his thoughts, to direct his attention to others, and so to push the investigation until the unconscious factors are fully brought into the light of consciousness. Freud has himself described the process in these words: "The patient talks, tells of his past experiences and present impressions, complains, and expresses his wishes and his emotions. The physician listens, attempts to direct the patient's thought processes, reminds him, forces his attention in certain directions, gives him explanations and observes the reactions of understanding or denial thus evoked."[1] Later, on the same page, he remarks that the patient "will make the communications necessary to the analysis only under the conditions of a special affective relationship to the physician," the so-called "transference."

Now this is admittedly the method by which the facts of psychoanalysis are obtained, and an examination of its character seems to call for a considerable modification of the claim that psychoanalytical theory is based upon facts of observation. It is true that the theory is based on "facts," but these facts are not obtained by simple observation; they are reached by the employment of the method of psychoanalysis. This method intervenes, as it were, between the actual facts of observation and the prepared facts upon which the concepts are based, and it is of such a nature that the possibility of distortion cannot with certainty be excluded.

It has become a commonplace of psychology that the direction of thought, and its content, are influenced in a remarkable manner by affective and other factors, and it is clear that such influences are at least possible in the method of psychoanalysis. Before we can be satisfied that the communications of the patient, which constitute the facts of observation of psychoanalysis, are of the kind to which the term "fact of observation" is customarily

[1] Freud, *Introductory Lectures on Psychoanalysis*, English translation, 1922, p. 13.

applied in other branches of science, we must be satisfied
either that they are not distorted by the method of investigation employed, or that the degree and direction
of the distortion can be accurately estimated. An attempt
to apply this test to psychoanalytical research will be
rendered easier by a preliminary review of the knowledge
we possess concerning the potential sources of such
distortion.

The problem of the value of human evidence, that is
to say, the objective accuracy to be credited to communications made by one person to another concerning
matters of fact, aroused considerable interest amongst
psychologists in the earlier years of the present century.
It had been previously noted by historians that the old
standard whereby the moral character of a witness was
taken as the sole test of his reliability, and his statements
held to be accurate if his honesty was established, was
inadequate and misleading. It was apparent that, quite
apart from his honesty, his statements might be perverted by all kinds of factors of whose action he was
completely unconscious. Binet in 1900 called attention to
"the advantage that would accrue from the creation of a
practical science of testimony,"[1] and the suggestion was
enthusiastically taken up by Stern[2] of Breslau, who with
his fellow-workers carried out an immense amount of
painstaking research. Extensive experiments were devised, consisting essentially in the submitting of a pre-
determined experience to a number of subjects, and
subsequently obtaining from them an account of what
they had observed. The results were remarkable, and
showed conclusively that a witness's report of his experience, even when given with the utmost honesty and
conscientiousness, is rarely completely correct, and that
a proportion of the details, including even those of whose

[1] Binet, *La Suggestibilité*, 1900.
[2] The contributions of Stern and his school are mainly contained in
the two volumes of the *Beitr. z. Psychol. d. Aussage*, Leipzig, 1903-6.

truth the witness is absolutely certain, are erroneous. Thus in Borst's experiments only 75 per cent. of the items of which the witness was certain were in fact accurate[1]. If, instead of being asked simply to narrate what he had observed, the witness were interrogated with regard to details, accuracy was greatly diminished, though the range of facts apparently remembered was increased. This result is presumably to be attributed to the suggestive influence of the questions asked.

The mechanisms responsible for these perversions of memory were studied by observers who noted the influence of pre-conceptions, suggestion, and various other factors. Investigations of definitely pathological phenomena showed that extraordinary memory distortions may occur, such as the confabulations of the hysteric and the alcoholic, and the remarkable production of false reminiscences in the condition known as "pseudologia phantastica." Here the action of suggestion and other emotional forces was clearly demonstrable, and it was not difficult to show that the factors producing these exaggerated pathological effects were also active, though in a lesser degree, within the limits of the normal, and certainly capable of causing marked perversions. The conclusion to which all these various observations lead is that memory is an instrument whose reliability can be grossly disturbed by a multitude of factors, that no certain line between actual reminiscence and phantasy can be drawn except by some measure of objective verification, and that in the absence of such means a patient's statements concerning events of his past life can only be accepted with considerable reserve[2].

[1] Borst, "Recherches expérimentales sur l'éducabilité et la fidélité du témoignage," *Arch. de Psychol.* Genève, 1904.

[2] The value of human evidence, and the nature and action of the various factors responsible for perversions of memory are considered in detail in the author's "The Psychology of Rumour," a paper originally published in the *Proc. Roy. Soc. of Medicine* in 1916, and reprinted in the present volume (see p. 94).

Freud is, of course, well acquainted with the facts we have enumerated, and with the potential capacity for distortion inherent in human memory. He was, indeed, one of the first to appreciate clearly the difficulty of distinguishing between phantasies and genuine reminiscences, and it was this recognition that led him to abandon his original theory that the psychoneuroses were the result of psychic traumata. He discovered that in many cases the traumatic event, which was apparently responsible for the subsequent disorder, had in fact never taken place, and was merely a phantasy constructed by the patient's mind. In such cases the clinical picture was nevertheless essentially identical with that observed where the "traumatic" event could be objectively verified, and the conclusion was therefore inevitable that the specific causal factors could not lie in the event, but in the mentality of the patient. Freud held, however, that under these circumstances the objective validity of the memories produced by the patient was of relatively minor importance; he was concerned with the detection of intrapsychic forces, and for this purpose phantasies provided a material even more useful than genuine memories. Similarly, in the case of dreams, whether a patient actually dreamt as he related it, or unwittingly elaborated it on waking into an appreciably different structure, mattered but little to the work of interpretation, because in both cases the same forces were at work, and it was the discovery of those forces which constituted the problem at issue. This contention is applicable to the material produced during a psychoanalysis, and goes some way towards meeting the objections we have cited concerning the validity of that material. It is, indeed, a sound contention so far as the distorting forces arising within the patient's own mind are concerned. These would influence the flow of thought, but would by this very circumstance provide the necessary ground for their detection, and we should have no reason to deny to the flow of thought the title of "fact of observation," although the patient might be relating phantasies rather than actual memories. It is quite another matter, however, when the flow of thought is not influenced by purely intrapsychic factors, but by the intervention of the psychoanalyst. Under these circumstances the "memories" produced may be conditioned to a very significant extent by factors which lie entirely outside the patient, and the question of their value as indicators of the trends existing in the patient's mind assumes an altogether different aspect.

Moreover, the problem at issue is not merely concerned with memory. The whole direction and content of the patient's psychic processes are alterable by factors of the same kind as those observed in the case of memory. A lengthy investigation of a patient's mind means that one is no longer examining at the end of the investigation the object which one set out to observe, but an object which has progressively altered during the course of the investigation, and altered in a way which may have been largely determined by the investigation itself. This was the circumstance which vitiated absolutely and completely the painstaking conclusions drawn by Charcot and his school from the phenomena observed in the trained hysterics of the Salpêtrière. A perusal of the literature of double personality suggests strongly the existence of a similar vitiating factor, and in a case of this kind which I was personally able to investigate I had no difficulty in satisfying myself that much of the symptomatology observed was a direct result of the process of investigation employed[1]. It is not easy to avoid the conclusion that the method of psychoanalysis contains potential sources of distortion at least as great as those in the instances just mentioned. The preconceptions of the analyst, the particular moments at which

[1] Bernard Hart, "A case of double personality," *Journ. of Mental Science*, 1912.

he sees fit to intervene in the patient's narrative, the emphasis which he directs to certain features of the narrative, the point at which he deems a flow of associations to have reached a significant element, all these are abundantly able to produce decided alterations in the subsequent functioning of the patient's mind. It must be remembered, moreover, that psychoanalysis is a lengthy process, and that very small changes of direction in a long course may lead ultimately to a wide divergence. When the majority of the changes of direction tend to be in the same sense, as they are likely to be in investigations conducted by analysts trained in a particular system of beliefs and technique, then it is not surprising that the final pictures attained bear a close similarity. It may be noted in this connexion that, while the pupils of Freud confirm by their clinical observations the findings of their master, the pupils of Jung, working with weapons forged of much the same material and in a closely similar pattern, have no difficulty in finding ample clinical confirmation for the quite disparate tenets of Jung.

These objections to the reliability of psychoanalysis as a means of investigation are of a grave character, and make it impossible to accept the contention that Freud's theories are based on facts of observation, if the term "fact of observation" is given the significance which it possesses in other branches of science. Moreover, if the facts of observation are not beyond question, the conceptions and theories built upon them cannot be solidly constructed according to the canons of scientific method, and it is not possible to stamp them with the hall-mark of science unless and until the means by which they have been obtained has been shown to be trustworthy. The claim has been put forward that an inquirer can convince himself of the validity of the method of psychoanalysis by the process of having himself analysed, but clearly this claim can have no weight when the problem at issue is the determination of the reliability of the method itself. The attainment of an inner conviction is a phenomenon belonging to the sphere of religion, and without relevance to science; its existence may attest the spiritual or aesthetic value of its object, but not its right to be incorporated into scientific knowledge. The latter right can only be gained by rigid objective verification and demonstration, and not in the least by subjective convictions[1].

The claim that a person desiring to practise psychoanalysis must himself first be analysed in order to acquire the necessary technique is, of course, on an altogether different footing, and seems to be perfectly legitimate. It is perhaps also legitimate to require that the intending practitioner should undergo personal analysis to the end that he shall overcome his own "resistances," which would otherwise distort his judgment of the patient's mental processes. Clearly, however, this requirement can only be defended as a means of improving technique in a method already established, and it can contribute nothing to the demonstration of the validity of psychoanalytic method itself. On the contrary, the existence

---

[1] Freud has himself considered the criticism that the admitted influence of the physician upon the patient casts doubt on the objective validity of the findings of psychoanalysis, in his *Introductory Lectures on Psychoanalysis*, English translation, 1922, p. 378. He holds that this criticism is more satisfactorily refuted by the evidence of experience than by the aid of theory, and that "anyone who has himself conducted psychoanalyses has been able to convince himself numberless times that it is impossible to suggest things to a patient in this way." This would seem, however, to be a further resort to the "inner convictions" produced in the analyst as a ground for accepting the validity of his beliefs. It is of course possible to contend that in the sphere of psychoanalysis strictly objective verification is impracticable, and that a subjective verification is all that can be obtained, but such a contention would imply a decisive abandonment of the claim that psychoanalytic investigation satisfies the standards demanded by science. Freud's further arguments, relating to the verification afforded by therapeutics and the study of the insane, will be considered later.

of such a claim inevitably strengthens the criticism which asserts that the trained preconceptions of the analyst play a part in fashioning the material produced by the patient. This criticism receives a further justification when we note that the followers of Jung, whose theories differ fundamentally from those of Freud, make a similar claim that the practitioner of their method must undergo a personal analysis, of course by a member of Jung's school, before he attempts to deal with the problems of his patient[1].

In spite of the importance and weight of these various objections there are two points to be brought forward which serve to weaken their force. The first point is that psychoanalysis has a long history behind it, and many of its earlier discoveries were made by a process much less open to criticism than the method we have described in words quoted from one of Freud's later works. In these instances the intervention of the analyst was reduced to a minimum, and the "facts of observation" approximated much more nearly to the standard which science demands. A number of the more elementary Freudian conceptions and theories are solidly built upon facts of this character, they have attained a wide acceptance, and it is not unreasonable to regard them as established contributions to our knowledge. Moreover, it is necessary to emphasise that these comparatively elementary conceptions are nevertheless of the first importance, and have cast more light on the problem of nervous disorder than the work of any other psychopathologist, whatever verdict history may ultimately pass upon the later theories and practice of Freud. In view of these circumstances psychoanalysts might naturally claim that the elementary and earlier conceptions are the groundwork upon which their later methods are constructed, and that if the former are valid so also are

[1] H. G. Baynes in his preface to Jung's *Psychological Types*, English translation, 1923, p. xix.

these later methods. It is nevertheless difficult to accept this contention, because, although the margin of potential error in the elementary conceptions is relatively small, it becomes greater and greater the more an imperfect method is employed, unless it is possible to obtain objective verification by a frequent resort to the plane of phenomenal fact. This constant testing by an appeal to objective facts is a *sine qua non* in the development of any scientific theory, and we have seen that it is just this test which is lacking in the growth of psychoanalytical theory, because objective facts will not serve its purpose, but only those facts after they have been prepared by the method of psychoanalysis.

These considerations lead us on to the second point which serves to weaken the objections cited to the method of psychoanalysis. It is true that the facts are not of the order to which the facts of observation of other sciences belong, but this character appertains in some degree to all the facts of psychology. Except for the facts of introspection all other psychological facts are inferences. The only direct observation possible is observation of behaviour, of action, or of speech; in order to deal with these facts by the psychological method it is necessary to go behind them to the underlying subjective experience, which cannot be directly observed, but only inferred from the behaviour facts. In this way a new series of "facts" is obtained upon which the psychological concepts are ultimately constructed. This peculiarity of the method of psychology has been emphasised by Drever, who regards it as an inherent weakness, and one which dooms psychology to occupy always an invidious position in the scientific hierarchy, so that explanation of a particular series of phenomena by the concepts of another branch of science will always be accepted in preference to a psychological explanation, if both are available[1].

[1] Drever, *Instinct in Man*, 2nd edition, 1921, p. 4.

Moreover, although the facts of introspection are observed with a directness and intimacy greater than that attaching to the facts of any other science, yet they are by their intrinsic character incapable of objective verification, and we already know that they are subject to numberless sources of error unless they are made in a sphere in which emotional and other distorting factors are unlikely to play a part. It is objective verification which science insistently demands, and owing to the nature of its material psychology can only give an inadequate response to that demand. The objection on this score which has been taken to the method of psychoanalysis is therefore applicable to the whole sphere of psychological research. Nevertheless, there are degrees of deviation from the strict canon of scientific method. It may be true that every psychological conception rests upon facts which are separated from actual facts of observation by some measure of inference, but in many such conceptions that measure of inference is very small. In Janet's conception of dissociation, for example, the degree of inference is so slight that it may safely be neglected, and a similar statement is perhaps applicable to the more elementary Freudian conceptions, but in the elaborate later theories the actual facts of observation become more and more remote, and the degree of inference swells by progressive accretions until a satisfactory objective verification in no longer possible.

We are therefore compelled to regard the method of psychoanalysis as an imperfect weapon of investigation, and one capable of seriously distorting the facts which it elicits. Those facts, and *a fortiori* the conceptions built upon those facts, must hence be accepted only with reserve unless other sources of confirmation are available lying altogether outside the evidence furnished by the employment of the method itself. A number of such external sources of confirmation have been put forward, and these now call for some consideration.

The first confirmation proposed is that derived from the therapeutic results. Many of those who practise psychoanalysis formerly employed other methods, such as suggestion and persuasion, and they maintain that the cures now achieved are much more extensive and permanent. The conclusion is drawn that if a case treated by psychoanalysis recovers, this circumstance affords proof of the accuracy and adequacy of the method used. Unfortunately this argument has but little weight. In the history of medicine many structures have been built upon the fallacy of *post hoc ergo propter hoc*, and an appreciation of its significance and potency would no doubt shake other departments of medicine than that with which we are here concerned. In this department, however, its incidence and effects are peculiarly disconcerting and difficult to appraise. It is of course true that satisfactory results are achieved by psychoanalysis, but it is equally true that satisfactory results are achieved by many, indeed by all, other methods of psychotherapy, and by a multitude of methods which lie altogether outside the walls of orthodox medicine. Moreover, even if it be conceded that the cure is a direct result of the treatment, there remains considerable doubt as to the precise factors to which this result is to be ascribed, and it is possible that these do not belong to the essential structure of the method employed, but are merely vicariously associated therewith. For example, it is extremely difficult to delimit the results produced by faith and suggestion, and unless the activity of factors of these kinds can be accurately estimated, no certain conclusions can be drawn as to the efficacy of therapeutic methods into which such factors may enter[1].

[1] T. A. Ross, in his book, *The Common Neuroses*, 1923, pp. 7 ff., describes the various methods of treatment he has successively employed during his career as a psychotherapist, and points out that with each he obtained good results so long as, and only so long as, he himself believed in its accuracy and value.

The Freudian school does not deny that a factor of the order of suggestion enters into psychoanalysis; on the contrary, its existence is an essential part of their tenets. This factor is the peculiar affective relationship which develops between the patient and the physician, and upon it the "transference" processes, which are conceived to be a necessary part of the therapeutic action, are dependent. Freud expresses this affective relationship in terms of his libido theory, and believes it to derive its driving power from the psychosexual forces existing in the patient. He regards all forms of psychotherapy as involving this relationship, including those grouped under suggestion. He holds, indeed, that "A human being is... on the whole only accessible to influence, even on the intellectual side, in so far as he is capable of investing objects with libido,"[1] and that this capacity distinguishes the psychoneuroses which can be treated from those conditions, such as dementia praecox, in which therapy is impotent because libidinous occupation with an object, and hence the necessary affective relationship to the physician, cannot develop.

It is admitted, therefore, that an affective relationship, essentially identical with that underlying suggestive therapy, necessarily occurs in the course of psychoanalysis, and is indeed an integral constituent of the curative process. The psychoanalytical school maintains, however, that this affective relationship is not allowed to dominate the whole course of the treatment, as it is in the case of suggestive therapy, but that at a certain stage it is itself submitted to analytic dissection and finally dissolved. If this contention be correct it is clear that the accurate estimation of the results to be ascribed to suggestion, which we postulated as a necessary prerequisite before conclusions as to the therapeutic efficacy of psychoanalysis could be drawn, would immediately

[1] Freud, *Introductory Lectures on Psychoanalysis*, English translation, 1922, p. 378.

become possible. This contention is based, however, upon facts observed by the employment of the method of psychoanalysis, and its validity is entirely dependent upon the validity of this method. It can play no part, therefore, in a discussion in which the validity of the psychoanalytical method is itself the problem at issue, unless we are to be guilty of argument in a circle.

We must hence conclude that the argument from therapeutic results cannot provide the independent confirmation of psychoanalytic validity of which we are in search. It may be remarked here, however, that the opposing argument, which seeks to disprove psychoanalytic doctrine by the enumeration of alleged failures or harmful results, has still less weight. Quite apart from the inadequate and obviously biassed character of much of the evidence put forward, it is clear that here again the fallacy of *post hoc ergo propter hoc* is once more playing a potent part. To ascribe an unfortunate sequel to the method of treatment employed, rather than to the disease itself, assumes an exact knowledge of the nature and interaction of the complex factors involved which we are very far from possessing, and such a conclusion cannot be justified until that knowledge is attained. Moreover, even if it could be demonstrated that the sequel was the direct result of the method, this would but bear witness to the potency of the method, and it has frequently been pointed out that a remedy which is incapable of doing harm is hardly likely to be capable of doing good.

The second sphere in which it is alleged that confirmation of the findings of psychoanalysis can be obtained is the study of myths and folk-lore. It is maintained that there are to be found here human creations clearly exemplifying the processes which have been elicited in the individual by the method of psychoanalysis. A prodigious amount of research has been carried out in these fields by Freud's adherents, and the conclusions reached have been generally in accord with the principles of psychoanalysis. It is difficult to estimate the precise validity of these conclusions, because the actual objective facts observed in the research are admixed with a multitude of inferred facts of the kind peculiar to the psychoanalytical method, and anthropologists of other schools are by no means in agreement as to the deductions which may properly be drawn. We may admit, however, that the objective facts in this sphere do provide formidable arguments in favour of, at any rate, some of the findings of psychoanalysis.

The third sphere in which confirmation of psychoanalytic doctrine is to be found is that of insanity. The evidence here is perhaps more convincing than in any other field, because phenomena can be observed in the speech and actions of the insane which are entirely conformable to the principles deduced by the psychoanalytic method, and in which any influencing of the patient by the physician is excluded by the nature of the case. MacCurdy has emphasised the strength of this evidence in a passage which, at the same time, acknowledges the inherent weakness of the psychoanalytic method, and this passage deserves quotation. "Everyone knows that preconceptions determine observations very largely in all scientific work. We see what we are on the look-out for, and are blind to the unexpected. In psychoanalysis, however, this danger is augmented by the plasticity of the material which is largely produced in accordance with the theory of the analyst.... With this condition of affairs it seems extraordinary that Freud should, during the years when he was making his discoveries, have kept his eyes so vigilantly open for new factors and new unconscious phenomena, and that his general conclusions as to the content of the unconscious should be so accurately confirmed by examination of the insane who do not talk or dream to order."[1]

We may now endeavour to summarise our review of

[1] MacCurdy, *Problems in Dynamic Psychology*, 1923, p. 132.

the Freudian theories. The criticism which has been
levelled at the conception of the unconscious and other
of Freud's basic assumptions, on the ground that these
are impossible entities, is due to a misapprehension of
the nature of science and of the psychological method
of approach. The validity of these conceptions, as in
the case of all scientific conceptions, can only be determined by an appraisement or recapitulation of the objective facts, and the testing of the theories in the light
of these facts. The real weakness of the Freudian theories
depends upon the imperfections of the method of psychoanalysis as a weapon of investigation, whereby the
conceptions rest on inferred facts rather than on actual
objective facts. This weakness is inherent in some degree
in all psychological research, but it is graver here, because the deviation from observed facts to inferred facts
is exceptionally great, and introduces numerous potentialities of distortion. Moreover, these potentialities are
much increased by the circumstance that the method of
psychoanalysis may, owing to its peculiar nature, con-
tinuously alter the objective facts during the course of
the analysis. Nevertheless, many of the simpler conceptions are based on inductions in which both the
measure of inference, and the possibility of distortion by
the method of investigation, are both comparatively
small. Further, there are sources of confirmation outside
the method of psychoanalysis which at any rate give
some support to the conceptions. We may draw
the final conclusion that, although the theories of Freud
do not attain the standard demanded by the canons of
science, some of his conceptions approximate very nearly
to that standard, and perhaps as nearly as any psychological conception can approach. A consideration of the
immense advantage to be gained from the introduction
of a conceptual psychology as opposed to a mere description of mental processes, together with a due appreciation of the almost insuperable difficulty of obtaining

satisfactory objective verification in this sphere, suggest that some deviation from the strict path of scientific induction must necessarily be allowed, if we are not to abandon all hope of progress. The danger of such deviation must always be borne in mind, however, and it must not be forgotten that subjective feelings of certainty in the followers of Freud are no substitute for the objective verifications which science must insistently demand. The solidity of the foundations is vastly more important than meticulous additions to the upper stories, and we may reasonably ask for every possible means of investigation to be directed to the method of psychoanalysis in itself, with a view to establishing its validity, and eliminating or controlling the sources of error which seem to be inherent in it.

The later publications of Freud, culminating in *Das Ich und das Es*, published in 1923, have not been considered. The keynotes of this later work may perhaps be said to be an alteration in the direction of inquiry from the libido to the ego, an attempt to analyse and define the properties of the latter, and various speculations concerning the fundamental forces of the mind. None of this work could be made intelligible without entering into a degree of detail quite impossible here. For our present purpose it will suffice to note that the investigations do not essentially alter the earlier findings, but superimpose additional stories upon the older building, so that their validity is necessarily dependent upon that of the underlying structure. A further ground for criticism, however, may be mentioned. The later work of the Freudian school with its minute dissection of the libido and the ego into constituent parts, which combine and interact in various ways, introduces a mass of conceptual entities which approximate in their form to those of chemistry and physics[1]. Now it cannot be

[1] Dr Ernest Jones, for example, formulates the following theory of the nature of suggestion and autosuggestion in his paper "The Nature of Autosuggestion," *Brit. Journ. of Med. Psychol.* 1923,

questioned that conceptual entities of this type can be legitimately employed if a stringent relationship to observed fact is rigidly maintained, but when they are reached by the extensive use of a spatial and mechanical metaphor, which can only be applied in the sphere of psychology by the exercise of some ingenuity and force, it is necessary to bear in mind the dangers which beset the road. The construction of such conceptions may no doubt indicate that psychology and psychopathology are attaining the precision and exactness of the mechanistic sciences, but it must also be admitted that the philosophy of Pythagoras produced concepts which appear to be precise and exact, and we need to be very sure in which of these fundamentally different directions we are travelling. The essential criterion lies in the relationship to the plane of observed facts. The concepts of mechanistic science are verifiable by a constant dipping to the level of experience and experiment, the speculations of Pythagoras can be submitted to no such test. The psychoanalytic school of course claim that this criterion is applicable to their work, and that the conceptions they put forward are legitimately built upon clinical observa-

p. 208: "Suggestion is essentially a libidinal process: through the unification of the various forms and derivatives of narcissism the criticising faculty of the ego-ideal is suspended, so that ego-syntonic ideas are able to follow unchecked the pleasure-pain principle in accordance with the primitive belief in the omnipotence of thought. Such ideas may either develop to their logical goal (beliefs, judgments, etc.), or regress to their sensorial elements (hallucinatory gratification). The essential part of the unification in question is that between the real ego and the ego ideal. The condition under which it takes place is that the repressed allo-erotic impulses are to be renounced. This is made possible by a regression of their libido in the direction of auto-erotism, which results in a further reinforcement of the narcissism. If the primary narcissism has been released and reanimated directly, by concentration upon the idea of self, the process may be termed auto-suggestion; if it has been preceded by a stage in which the ego ideal is resolved into the earlier father ideal the process may be termed heterosuggestion."

tions. We are therefore led back again to the problem of the validity of the method by which these observations are made, and to the cardinal necessity of establishing that method, before we can feel any security in the many-storied structures which are now being built by its aid.

The genius of Freud has produced a profound effect upon the development of psychopathology. In addition to the orthodox school of psychoanalysis, which follows more or less rigidly the path sanctioned by its founder, a multitude of other investigators have been materially influenced by Freud's conceptions. Many of these investigators are prepared to travel a certain distance with Freud, although they refuse to accept his views in their totality. Others incorporate individual psychoanalytic conceptions in theories mainly built on other lines, as we have seen to be the case with certain persuasionist and suggestionist practitioners of the present day. None of these writers call for individual mention here, as they do not add anything essentially new to the principles we have already discussed, but merely adopt an eclectic attitude with regard to them. Two schools of thought, however, must be specifically considered, because, although they were both founded by men who were originally followers of Freud, they have now radically diverged from the orthodox path of psychoanalysis. These are the schools of Adler and of Jung.

Adler's views bear a broad general resemblance to the earlier Freudian theories from which they emerged, except that he finds the driving forces responsible for the neuroses and other mental phenomena, not in the sphere of sex, but in the will to power[1]. The precise character of these conceptions cannot be discussed here, but it may

[1] Adler's theories were originally developed in *Studie über Minderwertigkeit von Organen*, 1907, and *Über den nervösen Charakter*, 1912, both of which have been translated into English. A number of later works have since appeared, including *Individual Psychology*, English translation, 1925.

be noted that the method of investigation employed and the validity of the conclusions reached are open to all the objections which we have brought forward in the case of the psychoanalytical theories proper. It need only be remarked that the doubts we have expressed as to the scientific trustworthiness of the method of psychoanalysis cannot but bo onhanced when we observe the remarkably discrepant results achieved by it in the hands of men who start with different preconceptions.

Jung's work is of very great interest and importance. Its chief tenets may be described as follows: a denial of the paramount significance of sex, and the substituting of the exclusively sexual libido of Freud by an undifferentiated libido having the significance of a general psychic energy, and capable of expressing itself through any channel of human interest and endeavour; the doctrine that the unconscious includes a collective element common to the race in addition to its personal content; a theory of the psychoneuroses which, although it accepts the Freudian view that the basis of these disorders lies in intrapsychic conflict, radically differs therefrom in its interpretation of the forces engaged and their mode of action. Finally, there is in Jung's conceptions a significant change in the general attitude and in the angle of attack. He insists that a simple reduction of mental processes to their causal elements is inadequate, and that they can only be understood if their teleological and prospective significance is taken into account; and he holds that the symbols found in dreams and elsewhere are not merely "a sign of something repressed and concealed, but at the same time an attempt to comprehend and to point out the way of the further psychological development of the individual."[1]

---

[1] The later developments of Jung's thought will be found in his *Collected papers on Analytical Psychology*, English translation, 2nd edition, 1917; *Psychology of the Unconscious*, English translation, 1916; *Psychological Types*, English translation, 1923.

To consider the scientific validity of these various views would clearly be a formidable task, but we are fortunately relieved of the necessity of undertaking it by Jung's frank admission that his work does not satisfy the canons of science[1]. This admission is based partly on the contention that "purpose" cannot be included in the structure of science, because it is opposed to the principle of causality upon which scientific method necessarily depends. We have seen that this contention is disputable, that "purpose" can be included in causality in a wider sense, and that a purposive psychology can therefore be built within the method of science, although it cannot contain the reversible sequences of mechanistic science[2]. Apart from this point, however, Jung's methods are certainly in some measure extra-scientific, and indicate a reversion to that admixture of psychology with the viewpoints of philosophy, ethics, and religion, which characterised the speculations of older days. But it is important to note that the admixture here is not due to a confusion of thought or a failure to distinguish the functions of the various disciplines, but is deliberately selected as likely to add most to human knowledge.

This is the chief interest of Jung's work in relation to the subject of the present lectures. It expresses a revolt against the view that the method of science must be the paramount arbiter of human knowledge, and attempts to substitute for this the principle that, while human life and thought cannot be explained by concepts belonging to science, they can be explained by other modes of attack. The question at issue is no longer whether psychology is capable of achieving the necessary standards of science, but whether science is capable of fulfilling the requirements of psychology. This is a bold step, but there is a good deal to be said in its justification. MacFie

[1] Jung, *Analytical Psychology*, English translation, 2nd edition, 1917, p. xv.
[2] Cf. Lecture II, p. 40

Campbell has remarked: "We are too much accustomed
to think that there is only one correct way of dealing
with experience, and that the angle, from which we
personally come to experience, is the only one from which
it can be approached....The results and methods of
others we are liable to see only as mistake and error,
instead of merely as another way of dealing with experience."[1] It is here that the essential antithesis lies
between the doctrines of Jung and of Freud. While Jung
abandons science as incapable of dealing adequately
with the problems of psychology, Freud strives to keep
within its bounds. Moreover, in Freud's later work his
conceptions approximate in their form to those of the
mechanistic sciences, and the divergence from the point
of view of Jung becomes still more marked. We have
seen that there is some reason to question how far Freud
has achieved success in this aim, but, even if success be
admitted, Jung's attitude is a reminder that the method
of science may conceivably not be the only weapon
whereby the field of psychology can be attacked, and
that it may ultimately prove to be an ill-adapted and
essentially inadequate weapon. Dr T. W. Mitchell, in a
review of Freud's *Beyond the Pleasure Principle*, says:
"The pessimism which hangs like a cloud over the whole
of this essay is perhaps the inevitable outcome of a belief,
however achieved, in a mechanistic theory of life; and
perhaps the criticism which will, in the end, invalidate
Freud's arguments, may come, not from those who dispute the accuracy of his deductions, but from those who
question the fundamental assumption on which all his
reasoning rests—the assumption that all the phenomena
of life and mind can be interpreted in terms of the
physical sciences."[2]

[1] MacFie Campbell, "On recent contributions to the study of
the Personality," published in *Problems of Personality (Studies in
honour of Morton Prince)*, 1925, p. 74.

[2] T. W. Mitchell, *Brit. Journ. of Med. Psychol.* 1923, p. 243.

Now no scientist with any appreciation of the real nature of science as a mere weapon for attacking and controlling our experience, and not as a unique road to the attainment of absolute knowledge, would contend that this is the only conceivable weapon, or that other weapons may not prove to be ultimately more effective. He may reasonably hold, however, that at present it is the only weapon which he feels he can trust, that the other methods hitherto proposed lead him into a sea of divergent speculations in which he can find no solid ground whereon to build with surety, and that he is at least justified in pushing the method of science to its limits in the field of psychology, before he consents to abandon a mode of attack which has succeeded in the past few centuries in giving us a control of our experience incomparably greater than anything before achieved.

Whether or no it will ultimately be shown that a psychology founded on the method of science is inadequate, it is at least desirable that we should know with certainty when we are employing that method and when we are going beyond it. The aim of the foregoing criticism of Freud's work has been to set out in broad lines the respects in which it satisfies the canons of scientific validity, and those in which it appears to fall short thereof. The reproach will rightly be levelled at this criticism that it attains to no certain point of acceptance and rejection, and it can only be pleaded in justification that this picture of benevolent scepticism portrays faithfully the stage in the road of conviction to which the mind of the writer has succeeded in travelling.

These various considerations lead us to a further point. The spheres of medicine and science are not quite the same, however much we may strive to identify them. On the one hand medicine is partly an art, and on the other hand its essential goal is therapeutic result, and not the acquirement of pure knowledge. Therapeutics has a normative aim, and normative aims cannot be fitted squarely into the structure of positive science. Hence medicine cannot afford to submit itself entirely to the narrow and rigid limits of science, but must demand a greater degree of freedom. In therapeutics it is justifiable to act on hypotheses which lack full or perhaps any scientific validity. Medicine has always claimed this right in very liberal measure, and the prin- ciple must be applied to the sanctioning as therapeutic procedures of psychoanalysis and the many variants and derivatives of psychoanalysis, until our knowledge is commensurate with the task of giving or denying to them an assured place in our professional armoury.

Finally, a word may be said concerning the actual and potential relationships of psychopathology to the other avenues of attack which seek to penetrate the field of medicine. In the first lecture it was pointed out that, while psychology must insist upon the privilege of for- mulating its own concepts and extending these so far as they are found to be useful in the explanation of human life and behaviour, the possibility must always be kept in mind that these concepts may ultimately be capable of reduction to the wider concepts of some other branch of science. Just as the concepts of physiology may in the future be brought under the concepts of chemistry and physics, so may psychology be merged in a wider physiology, and psychopathology in a wider pathology. This complete merging may never be practicable, por- tions of experience only to be dealt with by psychological conceptions may "stick out," however far we may ulti- mately succeed in thrusting the major part of the phenomena of psychology into a physiological or chemical framework. We have seen, for example, that "purpose," which seems to be an integral factor in psychology, appears to be inherently incapable of incorporation into the structure of mechanistic science[1]. Nevertheless, as

[1] Cf. Drever, *Instinct in Man*, 2nd edition, 1921, p. 5: "... the psychologist finds in the psychical series important factors, which

each branch of science is justified in endeavouring to explain as much of our experience as it can, the aim of subsuming the concepts of one branch under the wider concepts of another branch is clearly a desirable one in the interests of the unification of knowledge. It will therefore be profitable to inquire how far such an aim has been achieved, or shows prospects of being achieved, so far as psychopathology is concerned.

We must confess that up to the present time but little solid progress in this direction can be reported, though innumerable attempts have been made to bring the problems of psychology and psychopathology under the conceptions of physiology. Most of these attempts have consisted, however, in the preliminary acceptance of a psychological conception, and a subsequent free translation of its terms into hypothetical nerve forces and nerve units, a process which seems to give ineffable satisfaction to certain minds, but which adds little or nothing to our knowledge and understanding. Other attempts have led to the construction of anatomical and physiological concepts built entirely in the air, without basis or means of verification on the plane of objective facts, and therefore without scientific justification or utility. Nevertheless something has been done, and vistas have been opened up along which prospects of considerable future progress may be discerned. One such vista has been offered by the development of endocrinology. It is not difficult to foresee a time in which the psychological conceptions of instinct and instinctive force may be partially reduced to the conceptions of biochemistry, and Freud has himself envisaged the possibility of certain of his concepts becoming ultimately capable of interpretation in biochemical terms. In the present state of

have, and can have, no analogue in the physical series, as, for example, conscious purpose. It may be argued, therefore, that psychology will always preserve biology from being swallowed up by physiology."

our knowledge, however, all this does not take us very far beyond the realm of speculation. However desirable the merging of psychopathology in general pathology may be held to be, it must be admitted that the time for its consummation has not yet arrived, and that there is a field in which psychopathology can aid our understanding and our practice in a way not yet possible for physiopathology. So long as this holds it is more profitable, both for science and for medicine, that psychopathology should be allowed to march independently as best it can, rather than that general pathology should burst its legitimate bounds in a dubious attempt to incorporate phenomena with which it is at present unfitted to cope.

THE PSYCHOLOGY OF RUMOUR[1]

THE subject of "rumour," though at all times a fascinating field for the psychologist, possesses to-day an exceptional importance and interest. The prevalence of rumour during the War has furnished an overwhelming demonstration of the fallibility of human evidence, and has provided a mass of material which should yield a rich harvest to the scientific investigator. The aim of the present paper is to indicate the results which in the past psychology has already achieved in this field, and the bearing of those results upon the problems of the present day.

Rumour is a complex phenomenon consisting essentially in the transmission of a report through a succession of individuals. It may be provisionally regarded as the product of a series of witnesses, each of whom bears testimony to a statement imparted to him by his predecessor in the series[2]. The reliability of a rumour depends, therefore, upon the accuracy with which each such statement is transmitted, and ultimately upon the accuracy of the report furnished by the first member of the series, who is assumed actually to have seen or heard the event in question. This latter factor, the testimony of the actual witness of an event, is what the law terms "evidence," and it is clear that an examination of its psychology must precede any attempt to attack the more complicated problem of rumour.

The first scientific investigation of evidence seems to have been carried out, not by psychologists nor by jurists,

---

[1] Originally published in the *Proc. Roy. Soc. of Medicine*, 1916.
[2] It is necessary to emphasise the provisional character of this definition. We shall subsequently find that it is incomplete, and that it requires considerable modification (*vide* p. 111).

but by historians. The methods of historians in estimating the value of evidence have undergone a considerable change in modern times. Formerly they accepted the moral character of a writer as the test of his reliability; if his character was known to be good then the statements which he made were held to be accurate. They debated whether their witness was honest or dishonest, whether he spoke truth or was deliberately trying to mislead for certain definite conscious ends. If this question was decided in the witness's favour then all his evidence was accepted. Now, however, the reliability of each individual statement is separately estimated. The moral character of the witness remains, of course, an important factor, but the historians also take into account every possible condition which may have exerted an influence upon the particular statement under examination: the source of the witness's knowledge, the time-interval separating him from the events in question, his views and prejudices, his profession, religion, and political party. They consider, moreover, not only whether the witness is deliberately lying, but whether and how far he is unconsciously perverting the truth owing to the action of the factors just mentioned. In recent years attempts have been made to codify the rules to be observed by historians in the estimation of evidence, and a considerable literature on this subject now exists, amongst which may be particularly mentioned the works of Ernst Bernheim[1].

Among professional psychologists the first definite step in the direction of investigating the psychology of evidence seems to have been taken by Binet[2], who in *La Suggestibilité* (1900) called attention to "the advantage that would accrue from the creation of a practical science of testimony." The suggestion was taken up enthusias-

[1] Ernst Bernheim, "Das Verhältnis der historischen Methodik zur Zeugenaussage," *Beitr. z. Psychol. d. Aussage*, Leipzig, 1903.
[2] Binet, *La Suggestibilité*, Paris, 1900.

tically by Stern, of Breslau. Stern[1] founded a school of experimental psychology whose energies were almost entirely devoted to the psychology of evidence. Their work was in the main experimental, and they carried out a prodigious amount of painstaking research. One can make no attempt to give any adequate account of this work here, but it will be of interest to describe the general methods employed, and to give a short résumé of the principal conclusions reached.

The methods adopted all consist essentially in submitting a pre-determined experience to a number of subjects, subsequently obtaining from the latter a report of what they have experienced, comparing the reports with the original experience, and finally collating and evaluating the results thereby achieved. For example, a picture is shown for a defined period of time, and after a fixed interval each observer is required to give evidence as to the nature and details of the picture he has seen. The time-interval between observation and report may be varied from nothing to several weeks. The report is obtained by two different methods—narrative and interrogatory. In the former the subject is asked to write out as fully as possible all he has seen. In the interrogatory method a number of questions are asked by the experimenter, designed to cover in their entirety all the details of the original experience. The subject is asked, for example, "Were there any animals in the picture?" "What colour were they?" The questions are carefully constructed and classified into simple inquiries devoid of any suggestive implication—e.g. "What is the size of the picture?"—and "leading questions" containing suggestive implications of various degrees—e.g. "Has the man a brown coat?" The interrogatory method corresponds essentially with the "cross-examination" of our law

[1] The papers of Stern at his school have been published in the two volumes of the *Beitr. z. Psychol. d. Aussage*, Leipzig, 1903–6, and in the *Zeitschr. z. angewandt. Psychol.* Leipzig

courts. Each detail of a report obtained by these methods is graded according to the subject's assurance of its reliability. The degrees of assurance generally distinguished are "complete uncertainty," "hesitancy," "certainty," and "attestation." "Attestation" means that the subject is prepared to swear to the truth of the evidence in question.

The most important general result of the experimental investigations conducted along these lines is that they upset in the most definite and complete manner two naïve views widely held by the laity: (1) that evidence given with the best knowledge and honesty is a correct reproduction of actuality; (2) that evidence which is shown to be false must be due to deliberate lying, or at least to culpable carelessness.

Experiment shows us that completely correct reports are not the rule but the exception, even when the report is made by a competent observer under favourable conditions. It must be clearly understood, moreover, that this statement remains true if only those details are taken into consideration of whose accuracy the reporter is certain. Borst[1] found in 240 reports only 2 per cent. of errorless narratives and 0·5 per cent. of errorless depositions—i.e. reports obtained by the interrogatory method. The average reporter, when no suggestive questions are employed, exhibits a coefficient of accuracy of roughly 75 per cent. In other words, only 75 per cent. of the items of which the reporter is *certain* are in fact accurate. Moreover, attestation does not guarantee accuracy. Although the number of errors in sworn testimony is considerably less than that in unsworn testimony, they may nevertheless amount in the former to as much as 10 per cent.

A detailed examination of the results obtained by these investigations yields a large number of interesting

[1] Borst, "Recherches expérimentales sur l'éducabilité et la fidélité du témoignage," *Arch. de Psychol.* Genève, 1904.

facts, of which the following may be selected for special mention: The effect of increasing the time-interval between the observation and the moment when the witness is called upon to give evidence regarding it, is that, though range and accuracy are both diminished, assurance is not equally affected, but shows a surprising constancy. This statement, rendered in non-technical language, means that, though the number of details remembered and their accuracy are both diminished by lapse of time, the witness's belief in the truth of his evidence is but little affected. From this it may be concluded that assurance, and readiness to swear to the truth of the evidence given, depend upon the "personal equation" of the witness rather than upon freshness of memory. A second interesting fact established by the experiments is that, if the interrogating method is employed instead of the narrative method, the range is increased but the accuracy is greatly diminished, that is to say, more details are remembered but fewer are truthfully reported. This is, of course, due to the suggestive influence exercised by the questions asked. The diminution of accuracy when definitely suggestive or leading questions are used is evident enough in adults, but in children this effect is very marked indeed. For this reason evidence given by children should only be accepted with the greatest caution; their range is small, their accuracy smaller still, while their assurance is relatively very high.

It will be seen at once that these experimental results are of very great practical value, and that they establish conclusively certain basic facts which are of fundamental importance to the psychology of evidence. Stern and his school, however, do not get much beyond this. Their work, except here and there, presents us with no dynamic view of the forces responsible for the facts they describe, no conceptions which enable us to understand *why* these things do and *must* take place.

We get some illumination in these respects, however,

from a third group of investigators, who approach the subject from a different point of view and with a very practical aim—the jurists. The lawyer must obviously have a considerable interest in the psychology of evidence, and legal authorities have from time to time during the past two centuries shown that they possessed at any rate some inkling of the principles ultimately laid down by Stern and the Breslau school. Jeremy Bentham concerned himself with the subject in considerable detail, and later legal writers have dealt with supposed perjuries and the danger of suggestive questions. The first comprehensive and detailed work from the legal side on the psychology of evidence, however, would seem to be that of Hans Gross, the well-known criminologist.

Gross[1] points out that the psychology of evidence involves, not only a memory-process and the question of the fidelity of that process, but also the processes of perception and registration which take place at the moment of the occurrence reported upon, and he holds that even more weight is to be ascribed to these latter processes than to the former. He lays stress on the personal equation of the observer, and shows that the same objective event may be very differently perceived by different observers[2]. What a man sees depends not only on what is actually presented to him at the moment, but on perceptual additions due to prior knowledge and interests. He tends to group an event egocentrically, to over-weight the factors which arouse his interest and to

[1] Hans Gross, "Das Wahrnehmungsproblem und der Zeuge im Strafprozess," *Archiv f. Strafrecht u. Strafprozess*, 1902.

[2] Gross points out that we do not actually see what happens in a moment of time, but a combination picture, grouped from successive moments, and the mode of grouping may be different in different observers. Thus, if an event objectively consists of *a, b, c, ...*, then one observer may perceive *abc, def, ghi*, another *bcd, efg, hij*, while a third may miss points and perceive *acd, fhi, kmo*. This conception seems to correspond with the "noetic form" of modern psychologists.

neglect others. This explains the paradox that an observer who knows nothing whatever of a subject may be a better witness, in a matter connected with that subject, than one who is an expert therein.

Another legal authority, Heilberg[1], brings forward some further considerations of great value. He points out the important influence exerted by events intervening between the observation and the report, and shows how the accuracy of a memory picture which is constantly brought up and discussed may be perverted, owing to the action of autosuggestion, external suggestion, and other factors, at least as much as a picture left in pure passivity. He explains by this principle the epidemic of false witnesses which so often occurs in the later stages of sensational trials. Heilberg, moreover, illuminates the path along which we must tread in our search for the psychological laws responsible for the perversion of evidence, in that he calls our attention to the influence exerted upon the witness by the solemnity of the court, the feeling that he occupies the centre of the stage and that his words are big with fate, and the consequent appeal to his vanity.

Some extremely interesting and stimulating observations are to be found in an article written by Stern in collaboration with his wife, entitled "Memory and Testimony in Early Childhood,"[2] and consisting essentially of a study of the gradually developing mind of their own child. The points which we desire specially to mention are contained in a chapter on "False Witness in Children." Here the authors develop the important proposition that between lies and genuine perversions of memory there exists an intermediate group of phenomena, to which they give the name of "pseudo-lies." The com-

[1] A. Heilberg, "Zum Aussagestudium," *Beitr. z. Psychol. d. Aussage*, Leipzig, 1903.

[2] Stern, "Errinerung und Aussage in der ersten Kindheit," *Beitr. z. Psychol. d. Aussage*, II, Leipzig.

monest variety of these pseudo-lies is the relation of some
fiction which the child represents as an event which
actually occurred. On one occasion, for example, a child
informed her parents, after a visit to the Zoo, that she
had stroked the bears, and became tearfully and stormily
insistent when the veracity of her account was called
into question. This, of course, is the phenomenon which
we term "phantasy," and which is familiar to us in the
day-dreaming of the adolescent. In the child, however,
phantasy is not sharply distinguished from reality, and
it tends to play with fictitious accounts of past events,
just as it plays with fictitious representations of the
present. "While reality and make-believe in the life of
the child are not yet distinct from one another, so also
are truth and falsehood not yet distinct." A similar
inability to distinguish truth from phantasy has been
noted by Cramer[1] in the case of imbeciles.

So far as I have been able to discover, Stern does not
seem to have applied these valuable observations upon
the forces at work in the child to the problem of the psychology of testimony in the adult, nor to have realised
that the adult is moved by precisely the same forces as
the child, though of course less blatantly, and with their
action modified by other factors.

The part played by phantasy in the psychology of
testimony has also been dealt with by the historian,
Ernst Bernheim[2]. This author has seen, moreover, the
close relationship between the mechanism at work here
and that underlying the evolution of myths and sagas, a
problem to which we shall subsequently return. Bernheim
also remarks on the influence exerted on the witness by
the impulse to assign satisfying motives and to round off
the story. When we pass from the question of testimony
to that of the transmission of a report through a number

[1] Cramer, "Ueber die Zeugnisfähigkeit bei Geisteskrankheit
und bei Grenzzuständen," *Beitr. z. Psychol. d. Aussage*, i, Leipzig.
[2] *Loc. cit.*

of witnesses—i.e. from the question of evidence to that
of rumour—the recognition of this factor becomes of
essential importance.

Now if we review the various facts elucidated by the
investigators we have so far considered, and endeavour
to group them into a coherent whole, we shall find that
our task will be greatly facilitated by applying to those
facts certain conceptions employed in modern psychology,
in particular the conception of the "complex." We shall
thereby be enabled, moreover, to obtain a considerable
insight into the mechanisms responsible for the phenomena whose existence has been demonstrated.

A "complex" may be defined as a system of related
ideas possessing a certain affective load, which tends to
produce in consciousness trains of thought leading in a
definite direction[1]. Thus we explain the circumstance
that two politicians will arrive at diametrically opposite
conclusions when presented with the same body of facts,
by saying that the train of thought is directed in the one
case by a Conservative complex, in the other by a Liberal
complex. It is held, moreover, that a complex may exert
its action without the individual himself being in the
least aware that his thinking is so directed. The individual may, indeed, believe the causes responsible for the
conclusion he has reached to be quite other than they

[1] "Complex" is defined here in a wider sense than that now
customarily employed. The current usage is to limit the term to
systems which are repressed, and therefore more or less pathological. It is held that for systems which are not repressed the
concept of "constellation," or better still "sentiment" in the
sense in which it is generally understood in modern psychology,
is sufficient. There are good grounds, however, for employing a
word which will connote a system with the properties described
in the text, whether that system is or is not subject to the accident
of repression. Moreover, A. G. Tansley, in a symposium on "Complex and Sentiment" published in the *Brit. Journ. of Psychol.* 1922,
has pointed out that Jung, who originally devised the term
"complex," did not limit it to definitely pathological conditions.
See also footnote on p. 181.

actually are. For example, each of the two politicians may honestly believe that his opinion is the purely logical result of a dispassionate consideration of the facts presented to him. The process of self-deception by which this erroneous belief is given a superficial plausibility is termed "rationalisation."

This conception has proved extremely fruitful in both normal and abnormal psychology, and we can derive considerable aid from it in our investigation of the mental processes involved in testimony. It will be convenient to divide these processes into three stages—perception, conservation, and reproduction—and to examine in each stage the effects that may be produced by the action of complexes.

Firstly with regard to *perception*. It is an elementary commonplace of psychology that in every perception an endogenous factor is involved. When we perceive an orange, our percept consists, not only of the extensive yellow sensation which is all that is actually presented to us, but of an indefinite number of other factors, traces of former muscular and tactual sensations for example, which are added thereto from the store of our past experience. An endogenous factor of another kind is also present, however, whose activity accounts for the fact that perception is a selective process, and not a merely passive submission to sensations. We tend to pick out from the material presented by our senses the elements which are for some reason interesting to us, and to perceive only that in which we are interested. We may express this process by saying that our complexes exercise a selective action upon our perceptions. Complexes may exert, moreover, an action which is not only selective but perversive, and our perceptions may not correspond with the objects actually presented to us. Thus we tend to perceive what we expect to perceive, to mistake the stranger entering our gate for the friend whose arrival we are awaiting, to hear the motor-car for which we are anxiously listening. We can explain in this way some of the evidence which was showered upon us at the time of the Russian rumour[1]. I conversed personally with a soldier who assured me that he had himself seen trains filled with Russian troops passing along the line where he was on guard, and he described to me the tall bearded men and the unusual uniforms. The effects of complexes are proportional to their emotional strength. Hence there is a very grave danger of perverted perceptions in times of great emotional stress, a danger which must be carefully taken into account if, for example, we are called upon to weigh the evidence of even eye-witnesses of scenes occurring during the storm of battle or invasion.

Passing on now to the second process involved in evidence, *conservation*, we find further mechanisms by which perversion may be produced. Our memory-traces of events we have witnessed are subject to simple forgetting, whereby elements may be lost whose omission materially alters the picture, and to active forgetting, the process termed repression, whereby elements may be dislocated from their normal position, or essentially altered in their character. The manner in which the unhappy experiences drop out of our memories of former holidays, and the illusory rosy light which so often shines upon the past, may be cited as examples of this latter mechanism. In it, of course, complexes play an important part.

In the third and final process, that of *reproduction*, there are yet other mechanisms tending to the perversion of evidence. Some are due to the suggestive power exerted by the personality of the examining counsel, and the form in which he casts his questions. Here belong,

---

[1] A widespread rumour in the later months of 1914 to the effect that Russian troops had been landed in Northern Britain, and were being rushed through England for employment upon the Western Front. It was subsequently proved to be entirely devoid of foundation.

also, those effects produced on a witness by the particular circumstances attending the giving of his evidence, which have been insisted upon by legal investigators. Among such circumstances may be mentioned, for example, the solemnity of the trial with its paraphernalia, and the "centre-of-stage" feeling of the witness. The most prominent complexes here in action are the grandiose or "self-assertion" group. Hence arises an impulse which drives the witness to say something effective, to round off the story, and to fill in gaps—in fact, an impulse to stage his evidence so as to satisfy the canons of dramatic art.

Closely associated with these latter factors is phantasy, which may be regarded as affecting both conservation and reproduction. Phantasy is produced when complexes, instead of trying to achieve their ends by influencing the world of reality, obtain a partial satisfaction by the construction in the mind of trains of imagery, in which the ends of the complexes are, in imagination, abundantly realised. A simple example is the well-known daydreaming of adolescents. Stern, in the paper on the child to which we have already referred, fully recognises the important part played by phantasy in the perverted testimony given by children, but there is, of course, no doubt that this factor is fundamentally important in the adult also, although its action is not so obvious and unrestrained as in the child. Ogden[1] has pointed out that the essential difference between phantasy and memory does not appear to lie in any definite peculiarity of content, for intrinsically they are not clearly distinguishable, but that it is largely the problem before us with its directive tendencies upon which the practical distinction rests. Hence it is easy to understand that complexes, which occupy so important a position amongst the directive forces of the mind, may introduce phantastic elements

[1] Ogden, *An Introduction to General Psychology*, New York, 1914, p. 123.

into a memory-content without the interpolation being detected by the individual himself. As examples of the effect of phantasy upon evidence taken from the sphere of law, may be mentioned false confessions and the often-noted appearance of false witnesses in the later stages of sensational trials. In everyday life examples are easy to find. Our alleged memories of the events of early childhood are often destitute of any but the smallest foundation in fact, and that lack of veracity in the recital of past exploits, in which a possibly undeserved pre-eminence has been attributed to the fisherman, is by no means to be regarded entirely as the result of deliberate lying.

Our understanding of the part played by complexes in the perversion of testimony will be deepened if we take into consideration the facts provided by pathology. We should expect to find here, of course, perversions which are more obvious and accentuated. This very accentuation, however, will enable us to grasp their essential character, and thereby to appreciate the presence, though in a far slighter degree, of precisely the same mechanisms in the normal.

For this purpose it will be convenient again to divide the psychological processes involved in evidence into the three stages of perception, conservation, and reproduction, and to examine the pathological variations occurring in each.

The pathological perversions of perception include hallucinations, illusions, and certain delusions of reference. All these are now generally regarded as being due to the distortion of perception by an endogenous factor, and this endogenous factor can be traced, in some instances at least, to the action of complexes, whereby processes dissociated for some reason from the main stream of consciousness are, as it were, projected outwards.

It is a little difficult to distinguish sharply between the pathological variations of conservation and reproduction, and they may therefore be considered together. Here belongs the well-known phenomenon of paramnesia, of which examples frequently occur in many varieties of mental disease. Such, for instance, are the alterations in the memories of the past produced by a system of delusions, and the confabulations of the alcoholic or general paralytic. Most interesting for our present purpose is, however, the condition known as pseudologia phantastica, characterised by the relation of fictitious reminiscences. The patient, with an air of entire verisimilitude, will give a detailed and often elaborate history of his past life and experiences, which investigation shows to be wholly imaginary. Dr Stoddart, in a paper devoted to the description of an extremely interesting case of this disorder, ascribes the symptoms to the presence of a morbid instinct for lying. I must confess that I do not find this theory very satisfactory. Such an instinct would presumably affect all the patient's statements, whereas in fact only certain statements are perverted, and the perversion is always in a definite direction. Dr Stoddart's patient, for example, whom I subsequently saw at Long Grove, did not lie as to whether she had had beef or mutton for dinner, but only in the construction of a fictitious past which presented her as a distinguished, influential, and exceptionally interesting person. In this case the confabulations were evidently elaborate phantasies, whose creation we must ascribe to the activity of grandiose complexes, and it seems probable that a similar mechanism always underlies the manifestations of the disorder. Such a conception, moreover, enables us at once to understand the obviously close similarity existing between pseudologia and the ordinary day-dreaming of adolescents. This latter analogy has been noted by Risch[1] in the course of a very valuable paper wherein five cases of pseudologia phantastica are described. He

---

[1] B. Risch, "Ueber die phantastische Form des degenerativen Irreseins (Pseudologia phantastica)," *Allg. Zeitschr.f. Psych.* 1908.

finds in all cases certain common factors, among which
may be specially mentioned an irresistible impulse to
confabulate, with the consequent production of a peculiar
feeling of pleasure, and a characteristic egocentric orienta-
tion of the patient's trains of thought, so that the patient
is himself always the hero of his confabulations[1]. The
patients, in their pseudo-reminiscences, keep fairly well
within the possible, and only the total bears the stamp
of fabrication. Unlike the ordinary liar, they are un-
troubled by exposure, and merely stimulated thereby
to further confabulations, or to some often ludicrously
inadequate evasion. One patient, for example, when his
story of exciting adventures in the company of a Russian
count was demonstrated to be entirely fictitious, merely
remarked, "But I have nevertheless often met Russians."
So far as I can make out, Risch seems to think that the
patient has a genuine belief in his own fabrications,
although he endeavours to distinguish the condition
sharply from dementia paranoides. It is, however, very
questionable whether such a belief really exists. The
reaction of the patient, if exposed, is quite different from
that accompanying the demonstration of falsity of a
delusion; the fabrication *can* be exposed, the delusion
cannot. It would seem that in the pseudologia patient
the condition, as regards degree of belief, is a half-way
stage between the entire absence of belief found in the
case of ordinary day-dreaming, and the full and absolute
belief accompanying delusions. This half-way stage is

[1] Risch points out that these fabrications are related not only
to the phantasies of the day-dreamer, but also to the trains of
imagery which occur in the novelist and poet. He considers,
however, that the patient plays the rôle of actor as well as that of
author, whereas the novelist and poet play only the latter. This
is, I think, a misapprehension of the psychology of the novelist,
who, in many cases at least, obviously lives in the characters
which he creates. As an interesting instance we may mention
Mr Arnold Bennett's *Clayhanger* and *Hilda Lessways*, two novels
in which the same scenes are described, in the first from the standpoint of the hero, in the second from the standpoint of the heroine.

difficult to define, but it is probably closely similar to the pseudo-lying observed in children, which Stern has so admirably described in the paper we have already mentioned.

Nearly allied to the phenomena of pseudologia phantastica are the well-known phantasies of hysterics. An hysterical patient under my care at University College Hospital presented a member of the staff with some obviously freshly cut chrysanthemums which, she said, had been sent to her by a relation in California. When doubt was cast upon her story, she endeavoured to substantiate it by the production of a forged letter purporting to come from the relation in question, in which reference was made to his gift. As a further example of hysterical phantasy may be mentioned the well-known false accusations of rape. The complexes underlying these cases are, of course, obvious.

The importance of the facts of pathology in considering the question of the psychology of evidence is clearly very great, for they serve to show to what an extent it is possible for testimony to be perverted by phantasy. At the present time[1] numerous examples of these more extreme perversions are occurring, and are playing their part in the propagation of rumours. We may cite the case of the Scottish nurse, which attained considerable newspaper notoriety in the early days of the War. A young girl produced letters purporting to come from a hospital in France, describing the death of her sister after fiendish atrocities had been perpetrated upon her. The story was made public and aroused widespread indignation and sympathy, promptly cut short, however, by the alleged victim herself, who announced that she was alive and well, and had never left the confines of Yorkshire. Investigation showed that the girl had written the letters to herself, and that they were obviously the productions of hysterical phantasy.

[1] I.e. in 1916.

It must be remembered, however, that these pathological cases are only extreme instances of the activity
of a psychological process which belongs to the fundamental structure of the human mind, that the steps from
the pathological to the everyday are easily graded, and
that the phantasy which is responsible for the bizarre
phenomena we have latterly been considering, is made of
the same essential stuff as the normal phantasies of the
child and the quasi-normal phantasies of the day-dreamer.
Hence it is easy to understand that this process in its
minor grades may play a part in the perversion of evidence given by average men, and that it constitutes a
factor which must always be carefully estimated when
that evidence has to be weighed. Recent history has
shown, indeed, that such perversions of evidence in
normal men may, under suitable conditions, attain a
growth hardly less luxuriant and phantastic than that
we have described in cases which are definitely pathological. Except for recent history, we should, I venture
to think, have unhesitatingly said that in normal people
perversions could not occur to such an extent, and we
should have drawn the line between normal and pathological far more definitely than experience has shown
to be actually allowable.

So far we have dealt only with the question of testimony, that is to say, the report given by a witness on
some event which he has himself seen or heard, or which
he has himself experienced, and with the perversions to
which his evidence is liable. Before passing on to the
larger and more complicated, but closely allied, problem
of rumour, we may pause for a moment and summarise
the position we have been able to reach.

We have found, by the test of experiment, that a
witness's report of his experience, even when given with
the utmost honesty and conscientiousness, is rarely a
completely correct reproduction of actuality, and that a
proportion of the details, including even those of whose

truth the witness is absolutely certain, are erroneous. We have seen that these perversions are dependent upon forces of whose action the individual himself is mainly or entirely unconscious, and that amongst those forces a prominent part is played by complexes. It has been indicated, moreover, that the perversions of evidence which occur in the sphere of pathology are due to precisely the same mechanisms, and the study of the gross and obvious effects produced in these latter cases has helped us to appreciate and understand the more restrained effects which are met with in the normal. Conscious perversion of evidence, or deliberate lying, has not been considered, although, in any complete work on the subject, a chapter on this and its psychology ought undoubtedly to be included.

Earlier in the paper we have provisionally defined rumour as the transmission of a report through a succession of witnesses, each of whom bears testimony to a statement imparted to him by his predecessor in the series. Now if this definition were sound and sufficient our task would be practically over. It would only remain to point out that at each stage of the series the testimony given would be liable to perversion in the manner we have described, and that the measure of the final perversion would be the sum of the perversions occurring at all the stages. There can be no doubt, however, that such a view would be narrow and inaccurate, and that it would fail to take into account many facts of the utmost possible importance. It is a commonplace of knowledge that a series is something more than, and different from, the mere sum of its factors. The circumstance that we are dealing with a multitude of persons, that rumour is a social and not an individual phenomenon, in itself introduces entirely new elements, and these elements must be examined and appraised. Moreover, there are other facts not in accord with our provisional definition. A rumour does not always arise as the result

of a succession of reports proceeding from a single centre
of origin, but sometimes appears to show a kind of
spontaneous evolution, growing simultaneously from
many distinct centres. Such a phenomenon suggests an
origin other than a mere succession of witnesses, and
reminds us of the development of myths and sagas,
wherein legends almost identical in their content are
evolved in widely separated nations and countries[1].
Here again are new factors requiring investigation and
analysis.

Hence, although the transmission of a report from
witness to witness is an integral part of rumour, it is not
the whole thereof. It is for this reason that most of the
experimental work on rumour hitherto attempted has
failed to produce much illumination. The experiments
have been limited to the serial transmission of reports,
and naturally no new facts have emerged other than those
already ascertained in the investigations on evidence.
Rumour is, indeed, so complex a process that experi-
mentation is difficult to devise, and we are compelled to
fall back upon the experiments provided by Nature.
Fortunately she has not been niggardly during the War.

We have said that rumour is a social phenomenon,
that it is something which occurs in communities, and
has particular properties owing to that very fact. It is
therefore necessary to take into account certain psychological principles relating to the behaviour of communities, and especially of that particular kind of community
which we call a "crowd."

The psychology of the crowd has aroused much attention during recent years, and several authors have dealt
with it at some length. The pioneer and the best-known

[1] This view concerning the origin of certain myths and sagas
has been developed by the Freudian school. It is disputed, however, by many modern anthropologists, who maintain that a much
greater part has been played by actual transmission than was
formerly supposed.

of these is Le Bon[1], and the last is Sir Martin Conway, whose *The Crowd in Peace and War* was published at the end of 1915.

Le Bon pointed out that a crowd behaves differently from an individual, and he ascribed to the former an entirely distinct type of thought. His views may be shortly summarised as follows: Whoever the individuals forming a crowd may be, the fact that they have become a crowd puts them in possession of a kind of collective mind, which makes them feel, think, and act in a manner quite different from that in which each individual would feel, think, and act were he in a state of isolation. A crowd is always intellectually inferior to an isolated individual, for it does not think rationally, but is swayed by the emotion of the moment. The type of thought it exhibits is, indeed, fundamentally different from the rational thought of an individual. Crowds think in images, and each image immediately calls up a series of other images having no logical connexion with the first, but associated only by analogy or some other superficial bond. Subjective and objective are scarcely distinguished, there is no logical direction of thought, and hence contradictory ideas may be simultaneously present. For a crowd nothing is too improbable to be accepted, and a suspicion transforms itself as soon as announced into incontrovertible certainty. The convictions of crowds always assume a "religious" shape, by which term Le Bon understands blind submission to a being supposed superior, inability to discuss dogmas, desire to spread them, and a tendency to consider as enemies all by whom they are not accepted. The dominating force responsible for all these phenomena is suggestion, to which the crowd is peculiarly and characteristically susceptible.

Conway proceeds on much the same lines, but he takes "crowd" in a rather wider sense than Le Bon, to include

[1] G. Le Bon, *Psychologie des Foules* (English translation, *The Crowd*, London, 1896).

every "set," profession, class, or other possible congerie
of people. In this sense it corresponds fairly closely to
the various "social selves" of William James[1]. Conway
regards the crowd as moved essentially by emotion, and
contrasts this with the "reason" which is only to be
found in individual thought and action.

All these observations are of great interest, both in
themselves and in their bearing upon our subject, for
crowds are without doubt the soil in which rumours
grow and thrive, and an accurate understanding of the
psychology of the crowd will probably furnish a key to
at least some of the essential characters of rumour.

Much of this crowd psychology, however, is not
altogether sound. The distinction drawn between the
individual and the crowd is too absolute and too artificial.
The doctrine that a member of a crowd exhibits intrinsically different psychological mechanisms from those he
exhibits in isolation, that he becomes, as it were, a
different species of animal, is crude and untrue. Crowd
psychology is not intrinsically different from individual,
it is simply the psychology of an individual in a particular
environment, to wit, the presence of other individuals of
the same species. Hence there is no more justification
for the establishment of a special crowd psychology than
for a "man-in-an-engineering-shop psychology," or a
"man-in-a-potato-field psychology." The difference is
merely one of environment, and different environments
produce different reactions, whether the changes in the
environment concern persons or things. The essential
psychological mechanisms remain the same, although the
presence of other individuals may accentuate some, and
retard or inhibit others.

The fault of the crowd psychologists is not so much
that they have misunderstood the psychology of the
crowd, but that they have misunderstood the psychology

[1] William James, *The Principles of Psychology*, 1890, I, p. 292,
and II, p. 412.

of the individual, and have failed to appreciate that the latter shows the same type of thought as the former, though in a less obvious form. Le Bon's view that personal interest is the almost exclusive motive of an individual's conduct is a crude Benthamite doctrine which we cannot possibly accept. The statement, again, that the conduct and thought of an individual are mainly directed by reason is opposed to the teaching of modern psychology. The emotional type of thought, which we have called "complex" thinking, holds with almost as much force in the individual as in the crowd. Genuine "rational" thinking is a comparatively rare phenomenon, and much of the thinking which we fondly imagine to be rational is in reality the result of non-conscious complexes, whose action we conceal from ourselves by a process of "rationalisation." The difference between individual thought and crowd thought is merely one of degree, due to the very favourable field provided in the latter for certain emotional factors, which we shall afterwards define. The distinction between rational thought and "complex" thought is, of course, very real, but the line of demarcation is by no means the same as that between individual thought and crowd thought.

Among the forces responsible for "complex" thinking, a prominent place must be assigned to "herd instinct," the action of which in the psychology of civilised man has been demonstrated by Trotter[1]. Herd instinct ensures that the behaviour and thought of the individual shall be in harmony with that of the community. Owing to its action the individual tends to carry out the rules of conduct which are sanctioned by the community, and to accept without question the beliefs which are current in his class. For the average man it determines his ethical code and all those opinions which are not the result of special knowledge. It must be clearly under-

[1] W. Trotter, *Instincts of the Herd in Peace and War*, London, 1916.

stood that herd instinct is a determining force for the
major part of our individual thinking, and that it is not
peculiar to so-called crowd thinking. It is a fundamental
part of the psychology of each individual man, because
every man is essentially a gregarious animal. Rational
thinking is the only sphere in which its influence is reduced to a minimum, and genuine rational thinking
constitutes but a very small part of our mental activities.
It can easily be understood, however, that in a crowd
the conditions are peculiarly favourable for the action
of herd instinct, and that under such circumstances its
influence is likely to reach a maximum. Opinions and
beliefs are hence accepted more readily, and with less
demand for logical evidence, than in the case of the isolated
individual, and we should for this reason expect to find
in the crowd some approximation to that entire abroga-
tion of rationality observed by Le Bon and others. Our
conclusion will therefore be that the distinction between
individual thought and crowd thought is not a fundamental difference of kind, but merely one of degree. Non-
rational thinking is a frequent phenomenon in both, but
it is more obvious and unrestrained in the crowd, because
the crowd presents conditions which are peculiarly favourable for the action of herd instinct, and herd instinct
is one of the cardinal factors responsible for the non-
rational type of thought.

With these conceptions at our disposal we can return
to the problem of rumour, and endeavour to ascertain
what relation it bears to the psychological forces at work
in the crowd. This relation has been admirably analysed
by Trotter in his *Instincts of the Herd in Peace and War*,
and the conclusions he reaches may be expressed as
follows: Circumstances which stimulate herd instinct
tend to arouse characteristic gregarious responses in each
member of the herd. An increased sensitivity to his
fellows is produced, and an increased tendency to be
affected by, and to identify himself with, their alarms,

hopes, opinions, and beliefs. We have just observed an example of this mechanism in the case of the crowd, where the stimulus to herd instinct provided by collecting a number of individuals together, leads to a rapid contagion of non-rational opinions and decisions. It may further be stated that the strength of the gregarious responses produced are proportional to the strength of the stimulus to which herd instinct has been subjected, and that when that stimulus is maximal the gregarious responses will also attain to their maximum. Now war is probably the most intense of all possible stimuli to herd instinct, and above all a war in which the very existence of the herd is seriously threatened. Hence we should expect under such circumstances a vast increase of all the characteristic herd manifestations, including an abnormal sensitivity to the opinions and beliefs of our fellows, and hence an abnormal prevalence and propagation of rumour. Trotter points out that war, in order to produce a maximal gregarious response, must be a really dangerous threat to the herd. The South African War, for example, was not such a threat, and correspondingly the activity and vitality of rumour were not very great. Again, the stimulus to herd instinct was at its maximum at the outbreak of war in 1914. One will remember the extraordinary camaraderie which then prevailed, and the changed atmosphere of the railway carriage and omnibus. Correspondingly, again, rumour was considerably more rife then than later.

When herd instinct is maximally stimulated, its action overwhelmingly dominates the mind, non-rational opinions are disseminated with prodigious ease, and the rational activities, with their capacity for cool criticism, are at a low ebb. In this way stories are accepted and propagated by people who, in a more normal state, would at once detect their inherent improbability or impossibility. To what an absurd length this logic-tight process may go was well shown by one of my servants, a not unintelligent girl, who inquired breathlessly one morning whether I had heard the latest news, to wit, that "one of our airships was up last night and dropped a bomb on Ilford."

We have thus reached a position which enables us to understand the nature of the soil in which rumours grow, and the factors which make it so fertile in time of war. The next problem which confronts us is the consideration of the causes immediately responsible for the origin and development of rumours, and the classification of the different kinds of rumours which we actually find in existence. To continue the metaphor, we have to determine the nature of the seed which must be cast upon the soil, and the different species of plants which thereby develop.

With regard to the first point, the answer must evidently be that the causes leading to the origin and development of rumours are all those factors which we found, in the earlier part of this paper, to be responsible for the perversion of evidence. Chief amongst these was the action of complexes, which were shown to be capable both of perverting the report of an actual occurrence and of creating fictitious evidence in the shape of phantasy. It is clear, moreover, that the kinds of rumours produced will depend upon the nature of the complexes underlying them. We cannot attempt here to make any exhaustive classification of these kinds, but the following groups may be fairly easily distinguished:—

(1) *Rumours directly connected with the Threat to the Herd.*—These are the product of the tension and anxious expectation induced in the herd whose existence is endangered, with the resulting perversions and phantasies thereby generated. Such, for example, were rumours of invasion, of spies, of Germany's big guns, giant submarines, and submarine transports. In some of these, other subsidiary factors were also undoubtedly concerned, particularly political bias, whose supposed burial under the stress of war was obviously by no means so complete

as we fondly endeavoured to imagine. This is very clearly shown by the attitude adopted towards such rumours by the newspapers which hauled down the old party labels in order to reappear under the new rival flags of government-baiters and government-apologists. The subsidiary complexes, which are thus enabled to find nourishment in this group of rumours, constitute a link which carries us over to the second group.

(2) *Wish-fulfilment Rumours.*—These are produced by the mechanism which is so familiar to us in both normal and abnormal psychology, the creation of a pleasant world of phantasy in which our desires and longings are abundantly fulfilled. As examples we may mention the rumours of Zeppelins brought down in the next county, of submarines sunk in the next bay, and the most won derful of all, the famous Russian rumour. Here again, of course, other factors play a part, some of which we shall mention subsequently.

(3) *Rumours due to Widespread and Fundamental Complexes.*—Certain complexes which belong to the essential psychological structure of every human being, and are therefore capable of being easily excited in large numbers of people, may, when an appropriate stimulus occurs, lead to the development and propagation of rumours. Such complexes tend to seize any likely material, and to build phantasies upon it in which they attain some degree of satisfaction. As an example of a rumour arising in this way we may cite the war-baby rumour[1], which seems to have owed its existence and growth to phantasies of an obviously sexual origin. In view of the eminently respectable character of many of the people who industriously propagated it, this rumour provides an interesting illustration of the indirect pathways by which the most efficiently repressed complexes will

---

[1] A rumour that the birth rate of illegitimate children had immensely increased, owing to the licence practised by, and extended to, the soldiers.

contrive to find an outlet. Rumours of atrocities, again, have probably at least one root in the sadistic and masochistic complexes which, at any rate in an undeveloped or repressed state, are more widespread than is generally thought. What may be called the instinct of cruelty seems to be an integral part of our nature, however much it may be concealed and repressed by our education and traditions. William James has clearly developed this conception in his *Principles of Psychology*, and he ascribes to the stimulation of this instinct the fascination which stories of atrocity have for most minds. It is easy to understand that phantasies built upon it may lead to the propagation of corresponding rumours.

Research has shown that fundamental and generalised complexes of the kind we are now considering, elementary complexes more or less common to the whole human race, play an important part in the development of myths and sagas, and it is interesting to note that the psychological processes concerned therein show a marked analogy with those responsible for the development of rumour[1].

There are certain peculiar aspects of rumour which merit special attention and analysis. The first of these is that curious impulse to pass on the rumour, to communicate it as soon as possible to a further person, of which the existence is a matter of common observation. A closely similar phenomenon may be noted in the case of wit, the impulse which we all feel to pass on the last good joke we have heard[2]. We may compare with it, also, that propagandism which Le Bon has noted in crowds, the imperative desire to spread their opinions and dogmas. It is possible, without pretending that the analysis is in any way exhaustive, to indicate two groups of factors which appear to underlie this impulse.

[1] Abraham, "Traum und Mythus," *Schriften z. angewandt. Seelenkunde*, Wien, 1909. See, however, footnote, p. 112.

[2] Freud, *Der Witz*, Leipzig, 1905.

The first group comprises the self-assertion or grandiose complexes, whose action we have already studied in the perversion of evidence. We noted there the desire to figure as a person of distinction, to occupy the centre of the stage, and to have the eyes and ears of our neighbours directed admiringly towards us; and it is clear that a similar feeling is obtaining satisfaction in the man who relates the latest rumour. It is instructive to note that the desire to achieve a position of importance in another person's mind is unquestionably present in cases of pseudologia phantastica, and Risch observed that his patients would only fabricate when assured of their hearer's interest. An interesting subsidiary effect of these grandiose complexes is the often observed tendency of the rumour propagator to bring the alleged events con stituting the material of the rumours as closely as possible into relation with himself. Thus, when spy rumours were rife, the propagator frequently assured us that the governess with the box full of bombs had been discovered in the adjoining suburb, or in the next street, or even in the house of his cousin. The pseudologia phantastica patient would have said that he had himself made the discovery in his own house, but in the more normal man the powers of self-criticism are still sufficiently active to inhibit a phantasy of this degree, but not sufficiently active to prevent the minor perversions we have described. The Russian rumour provided plentiful illustrations of this process, and there were few of us who had not an aunt, or a "friend in an influential position," who witnessed the travels of those wonderful troops.

The second, and probably the most important, group comprises the factors directly connected with herd instinct. We have observed that this instinct, when suitably stimulated, causes the individual to seek to identify himself with the herd, and to take a part in the promotion of the herd's welfare. If this desire can obtain adequate satisfaction, the longing and unrest produced by the promptings of the instinct are at once allayed. This effect is characteristically seen in the peace of mind and freedom from worry of the man who has, in a time of national stress, finally decided to join the army. The desire to identify oneself with the herd, to be "in it," and to play a part in its activities and strivings may easily be discerned in the propagator of rumour, and is clearly one of the factors underlying the impulse to communicate it.

Another peculiar aspect of rumour to which we desire to direct attention is the fact that it frequently exhibits a generic character—that is to say, rumour tends to assume a particular shape, which constantly appears whenever the circumstances are favourable. Thus when the Germans invaded France a rumour was immediately spread throughout Germany that the French had poisoned the wells. Similar rumours appeared on various subsequent occasions during the War, and have been current in former wars whenever an invasion has taken place. Of course, we are not in a position to say how much truth these assertions have contained, but their regular appearance at least arouses our suspicion. Similarly, rumours of atrocities have always tended to assume certain fixed forms. We may mention, for example, the rumour that many Belgian children were in this country whose hands had been cut off. Lastly, the best example of the generic character of rumour, whose very obviousness tends to prevent us appreciating its significance, is the circumstance that all the rumours during a war are concerned with the war.

We are unable to present any completely satisfactory theory to account for this generic aspect, but there are certain considerations which will at least cast some light upon the question. To begin with, the fact that rumours current during a war always concern the war, indicates that rumours will only arise in connexion with the subject which has bound the herd together, and stimulated to their maximum degree all the forces of herd instinct. Hence, in the case of war, they will tend to fall into forms which minister to the aggressive or defensive activities of that instinct, and these forms will naturally be fairly limited in number.

A further important factor in producing the generic character of rumours is the previously mentioned circumstance that the causal mechanisms fall into certain groups and thereby generate rumours of corresponding types. The last of these groups, the action of widespread complexes of a fundamental kind, would seem to be particularly important in this connexion. The identity of form shown by myths and sagas developed in remotely separated countries has been ascribed to their origin from complexes of primary importance which are common to the whole human race. It is clear that this generic character in myths and sagas is closely allied to that which we are now considering in the case of rumour, and we are therefore justified in assuming that the same mechanism is probably responsible for both.

One group of rumours, those concerned with atrocities, deserves special study in this respect. It is easy to discern in some of them the action of sadistic phantasies. Stories of rape and mutilation of women must obviously be sometimes due to this cause, and the circumstances of their origin would explain their stereotyped character. On the other hand, it is important to realise that sadistic complexes tend, not only to produce rumours of atrocities, but to express themselves in action, and to produce actual atrocities. Owing to the removal of inhibitions, always found in mobs, and certainly not least in a sacking army, we should expect these complexes to find in such circumstances an opportunity for active expression.

To this consideration we may appropriately add some concluding remarks with regard to the aims and limits of the present investigation. No attempt has been made to approach the interesting and important problem of the methods by which the perverted elements in evidence may be distinguished from those which are accurate. It is very obvious that reports are not always false, and that even rumours sometimes have a substantial basis in fact. No doubt it will ultimately be possible to devise criteria by which the wheat may be separated with certainty from the chaff, and the products of phantasy from the genuine results of observation. Law has long laboured to establish such criteria, and has evolved a procedure which is perhaps as satisfying as it is possible now to achieve. There can be no question, however, that this procedure is far from perfect, and that in it due weight is not given to factors which are obvious to the psychologist. We may reasonably expect that psychology should take a hand in the task, and provide the lawyer with information and with principles which will help him to improve the methods he now employs.

In the present paper, however, no such ambitious programme has been entertained, and the question of determining what is valid evidence and what is not has been entirely omitted. So far as rumour is concerned, the material selected has consisted solely of reports which have been subsequently admitted to be essentially false, because the problem aimed at has been the ascertaining of the psychological mechanisms by which such false reports come into existence. How far other reports —reasonably authenticated reports of atrocities for example—are true is a question of a totally different kind, and one to be solved, not by armchair speculations, but by a judicial investigation.

Even with these limitations the conclusions reached can only be regarded as tentative, for the subject and its ramifications are extraordinarily complicated and involved. I can only claim to have touched the borders of a vast field, and perhaps to have suggested some likely paths along which the future explorer may attain more complete results.

THE METHODS OF PSYCHOTHERAPY[1]

THE urgent problems presented to us by the war psychoneuroses naturally led to a greatly increased interest
in psychotherapy, and to the devising of many new psychotherapeutic procedures. So numerous and so apparently diverse have these procedures become that a
superficial glance at the rapidly growing literature might
lead one to suppose that the methods of psychotherapy
are legion, and that any attempt to collate and compare
them must necessarily be a task of great complexity and
difficulty. A closer inspection shows, however, that all
the available methods are ultimately dependent upon
the employment of one or other of three basic principles,
and that they differ only in the extent to which these
principles are combined, and in the particular technique
by which they are applied. These three basic principles
are suggestion, persuasion, and analysis[2].

Certain schools of thought profess to rely entirely or
almost entirely upon one only of the three, and name the
method they practise according to the principle selected.
Thus Babinski, and the many followers of Babinski who
have arisen in this country since the War, employ sug-

[1] Originally published in the *Proc. Roy. Soc. of Medicine*, 1918.
[2] A fourth principle should perhaps be included, namely "re-
education." This term is used to indicate two different psychotherapeutic processes. In the first place it denotes a process of
training whereby it is sought to modify a symptom, e.g. the
teaching of correct movements to a patient suffering from a func-
tionally disordered gait. In the second place it denotes the process
whereby causal factors, which have been elicited by analysis, are
modified or rearranged, so that they no longer produce morbid
effects. Re-education in the first sense is clearly a secondary
procedure, which is not entitled to rank with the three basic principles described in the text. Re-education in the second sense is
an integral part of analysis, and is included therewith for the
purpose of this paper (cf. p. 142).

gestion, Dubois and Dejerine advocate persuasion, while Freud, and the schools which have developed directly or indirectly from Freud, employ some form or other of analysis. In actual practice, however, these various schools do not confine themselves to a single principle, but in each case there is an admixture of other principles. Thus Dejerine, although a persuasionist, unquestionably uses suggestion to a very considerable extent, and the same criticism applies, though to a less degree, to Dubois, and to the practitioners of analysis. In spite of this fact each school tends to regard itself as the sole possessor of the promised land, and to treat its rivals as foolish mortals floundering uselessly in outer darkness. Now it is clear that, if we are to find our way through all these acrimonious discussions and disputes, it is necessary to determine precisely the nature and relationship of the three basic principles, suggestion, persuasion, and analysis, and the extent to which each of these principles is employed by the contending schools. The present paper is an attempt to progress some little way in the direction of this goal.

SUGGESTION

Suggestion is a widely used term, and is employed in medical literature as a convenient and satisfying explanation for all sorts and kinds of phenomena. Often, indeed, it is put forward as an ultimate and completely sufficient cause, much as if it were comparable in majesty and power to the law of gravity. Now this can only be justifiable if suggestion is a very exact conception, clearly defined and limited, and capable of precise formulation, and our first problem must be to determine how far the conception of suggestion fulfills these conditions. If we turn to the literature of psychotherapy we find that Dubois and Dejerine sharply differentiate suggestion from persuasion. The followers of Freud, on the other hand, hold that persuasion is essentially identical with suggestion, and that the method of psychoanalysis is absolutely distinct from either of them. A third school, again, maintains that psychoanalysis is merely an insidious and prolonged form of suggestion. Turning next to psychopathology, we find that Babinski regards suggestion as a sufficient explanation of hysteria, while other authorities ascribe the phenomena of "neurasthenia" to autosuggestion. Finally, psychologists tell us that suggestion is a normal process in the human mind, and that it is responsible for our religious and political views, our patriotism, caprices, and prejudices.

Now it is clear that something which explains hysteria and neurasthenia, and is a characteristic of normal health, which is responsible for our religion, politics, caprices, prejudices, and therapeutics, must either be a very inexact conception, or denote a factor so widespread and universal that it is useless to invoke it as a weapon of explanation. It explains everything and therefore it explains nothing.

It will be well, therefore, to investigate more closely the sense in which the word suggestion is used by these various authorities, to determine whether this sense is always the same, and whether the word is not sometimes used to denote processes which we already know under other names, and finally to inquire whether it is possible to formulate an exact conception to which the term suggestion may usefully be limited. A convenient starting point for this investigation may be found in McDougall's definition of suggestion as "a process of communication resulting in the acceptance with conviction of the communicated proposition in the absence of logically adequate grounds for its acceptance."[1]

Now the opening words of McDougall's definition, "a process of communication," immediately exclude a certain number of the phenomena which some authors bring under suggestion, but even with this limitation it is questionable whether the definition does not cover a

[1] W. McDougall, *Social Psychology*, 12th edition, London, 1917.

field so wide that the conception is of little use as a practical weapon of explanation. Most of our beliefs are held without any logical basis, though by the manufacture of rationalisations we endeavour to find such a basis when our beliefs are attacked, and we are constantly accepting propositions in the absence of logical grounds for their acceptance. The mind of man moves so frequently and universally along this road that to cite the process as an explanation of some particular phenomenon is hardly more satisfying than to explain the peculiar features of some animal or plant by the existence of an atmosphere. To begin with, if we adopt as a reasonable measure of "acceptance with conviction" our preparedness to act upon an idea, it may be said that every communicated idea tends to be accepted with conviction, provided that it does not conflict with other ideas. If it is announced to me that dinner is ready, I accept the proposition, and proceed to move into the dining room without instituting an inquiry into the logical basis of the assertion, unless the announcement is made at a time when I am normally expecting to go to bed. This is the process termed "simple communication," and there is no need to invoke any special function of suggestibility to explain its action. Such a process would appear to be all that is necessary to account for certain of McDougall's conditions favouring suggestibility, "lack of organised knowledge" for example. The acceptance by an uneducated man of a proposition patently impossible to anyone with special knowledge of the subject, is psychologically identical with my acceptance of the proposition that dinner is ready. When, however, a communicated idea is accepted when there are or should be conflicting ideas present, an obviously different process has come into action. If I am informed that one of my friends is playing golf, and I believe this assertion in spite of the fact that this same friend is sitting by my side, then clearly we are confronted with a phenomenon into which some other factor than simple communication must enter. This other factor is evidently a neglect or inhibition of ideas which are incompatible with the communicated idea. The first amendment to McDougall's definition which we shall therefore venture to propose is that the term suggestion should only be applied where such a neglect or inhibition of conflicting ideas is present. When, indeed, the phenomenon is due merely to neglect, the psychological process is so essentially different from that which underlies inhibition, that it would probably be advantageous to exclude it from the conception of suggestion. If, for example, we accept a proposition when we are fatigued which we should not so accept in our normally vigorous state, this occurs because fatigue has lessened the integrative capacities of our mind, and conflicting ideas are not brought into contact with the proposition which they would otherwise destroy. The process here is psychologically almost identical with the simple communication already described, and essentially similar to the acceptance by an uneducated man of a proposition which is in fact impossible. It would seem advisable, therefore, to reduce the limits of suggestion still further, and to confine it to those cases where there is an actual inhibition of conflicting ideas. This reduction brings suggestion into an interesting relation to attention, for in the latter there is an inhibition of irrelevant ideas, whereas in the former there is an inhibition of relevant ideas. The comparison opens up a promising avenue for speculation, but it would lead to fields outside the scope of this paper, and cannot be pursued further here.

If it is agreed that the essential process in suggestion consists in an inhibition of conflicting ideas and the resultant acceptance with conviction of a proposition based on illogical or non-logical grounds, we may next inquire whether this is a process with which we are already familiar under other names. A little consideration will show that we are very familiar with this process,

and that it has received many other names. It is the
process which I have called elsewhere "thinking due to
the action of a complex" as opposed to "rational
thinking"; it occurs whenever our stream of consciousness is directed by emotional or instinctive forces, and
it is responsible unquestionably for most of the movements of our mental machinery. The lover does not
fervently believe in the perfections of his lady because
he has logically deduced those perfections from the facts
at his disposal, but because all his thoughts and perceptions are twisted in a definite direction by the emotional
systems which constitute his love, and against that
directive force all the logic in the world is impotent.
Many of the beliefs and opinions of the normal man are
due to mechanisms similar in kind, though less grossly
obvious. It may be said, indeed, that the greater part
of our thoughts and activities are due to forces of which
we may or may not be conscious, but which are assuredly
not logical in character. Logic plays a part in directing
the minor currents in the stream, but the power which
drives the stream and determines its main course origi-
nates in emotional systems analogous to that which we
see in action in the lover. The effect of such an emotional
system is to throw into the stream of consciousness ideas
belonging to the system, to reinforce currents in harmony
with it, and to inhibit currents which are incompatible
or in conflict with the goal which it is trying to achieve.
These emotional systems are known by many names—
bias, prejudice, intuition, and so forth—but their action
is the same in each and every case, the forcing of the
stream of consciousness into a direction which will subserve the goal of the system, and the inhibition of all
ideas and tendencies which would conflict with that goal.
Now this action is precisely that which we have seen to
be characteristic of suggestion, and it will immediately
be clear that suggestion is merely a particular example
of the activity of an emotional system of the kind de-

scribed. To use the terminology which I have employed elsewhere, suggestion is a variety of "complex thinking."[1] How large a variety it constitutes is a matter of definition and arbitrary limitation. But its utility as a weapon of explanation obviously depends on the preciseness of the definition and the narrowness of the limitation, for if we make the conception so wide that it practically includes all types of "complex thinking," it will also include most of the mental activity of man, and its value as an explanation of some particular phenomenon will be almost negligible.

These considerations enable us to understand the apparently discrepant views as to the nature and action of suggestion held by the various authorities whom we have quoted. The discrepancies are due to the wider or narrower limits assigned to the concept of suggestion by each authority, and in part also to the absence of any clear-cut concept, or of any definite limits. While in some cases suggestion is regarded as including the whole sphere of "complex thinking," in others it is narrowed down to include only hypnosis and closely allied phenomena, and between these two extremes every intermediate grade may be found. Those who explicitly or implicitly embrace the first extreme interpretation, and who bring under the head of suggestion every mental process due to the action of an emotional factor, naturally explain a vast number of phenomena thereby, but factors of this kind are so universal that the explanation is correspondingly unsatisfying and incomplete. The explanation is true enough so far as it goes, but it does not go far enough to be of any practical use. If our knowledge is to be advanced we require to know what is the particular

---

[1] *Vide* the author's *Psychology of Insanity*, Cambridge University Press, chap. v. "Complex" is used therein in a more extended sense than that generally given to it, and indicates any affective system capable of directing and influencing the stream of consciousness. See footnote, p. 102.

emotional factor involved, and what are the precise circumstances of its operation. A perusal of the literature makes it very clear, indeed, that the indiscriminate use of the word suggestion in these cases is altogether pernicious, because too often it is regarded as a completely satisfying explanation, and the necessity of making further inquiries is entirely neglected.

It is evident, then, that if the conception of suggestion is to be practically useful it must be narrowed down to limits which will mark off a definite variety of "complex thinking," and which will not include any and every variety to which the word has been hitherto loosely applied. These limits will naturally be a matter for arbitrary selection, but it will be agreed that they should be so fashioned as to include within their boundaries those processes to which the word suggestion is universally applied, and only such other processes as can be shown to be closely allied thereto. In this way the common signification of the word will be preserved as nearly as possible. Now the processes which are universally regarded as typical instances of suggestion are the phenomena which occur in hypnosis, and the allied phenomena which are capable of being produced in the waking or normal state, and if we are to find an exact conception of suggestion it must be sought by an investigation of the essential features of these phenomena. In the typical instances in question a proposition is explicitly or implicitly stated by one person, and is accepted with conviction by another person, and it would probably be best to apply the term suggestion only to those cases where this direct relation between persons exists. This limitation is, in fact, partly but not completely implied by the opening words of McDougall's definition, "a process of communication." The amended definition of suggestion resulting from these various considerations would therefore read "a process of communication whereby a proposition is communicated by one person to another and

is accepted with conviction by the latter in the absence
of logically adequate grounds for its acceptance, and
owing to the fact that conflicting processes which are or
should be present are inhibited."[1]

It is evident that even this amended definition does
not give us a conception with sharply cut limits, for it is
easy to adduce a whole series of instances linking up the
typical examples of suggestion to almost any and every
variety of "complex thinking." If we are to establish a
sharply cut conception, it must be shown that in each
case where a proposition is accepted in this manner the
acceptance is due to the action of one particular psychological mechanism, and we may next inquire how far it
is possible to accomplish this.

Now in all cases of "complex thinking" the essential
feature of the process is that the stream of consciousness
is directed by a force which we have loosely described
as an "emotional system." Although these "emotional
systems" may apparently be of all sorts and kinds, it will
be found on analysis that they all derive their propulsive
and directive power from the incorporation within them
of one or more of the great instinctive forces of the mind.
The demonstration of this vastly important fact is the
noteworthy achievement of McDougall's work on social
psychology. If all "complex thinking" is due to the
action and interaction of instinctive processes, then suggestion, which is only a variety of "complex thinking,"
must also be dependent on forces of this character. Now
if it could be shown that suggestion, in the limited sense

---

[1] Dr Ernest Jones (*loc. cit.*) points out that the intellectualistic
definition of suggestion as a process leading to acceptance with
belief is inadequate, and omits a feature which Lipps and Janet
have emphasised, namely that the characteristic of suggestion is
not the mere arousal of an idea, but the further effects produced
by the idea when it is so aroused. Lipps holds, however, that these
further effects are the normal consequence of the arousal of an
idea, provided that opposing ideas are inhibited, and they would
therefore be implied in the definition proposed above.

we have proposed, owes its effects to certain particular instincts, or to a definite combination of instincts, we might then be able to formulate the exact conception of which we are in search. Several attempts have, in fact, been made to explain the process of suggestion by the action of such particular instincts or their combination. McDougall[1] ascribes it to the interaction of the instincts of self-assertion and self-abasement. Trotter[2] practically identifies suggestion with herd instinct, while Freud and his followers[3] maintain that the motive force is provided by the sex instinct. Space will not permit of a detailed examination of these various views, but it may be said that none of them is entirely satisfactory, and none of them provides the clear-cut conception we need. The evidence would seem to indicate, indeed, that the phenomena commonly ascribed to suggestion are not due to the action of any one instinct or combination of instincts, but that the motive force may be derived from different sources in different cases.

The conclusion to be drawn from these considerations is that, even within the narrow limits with which we have attempted to circumscribe it, suggestion is not a well-defined conception capable of affording a complete explanation of any phenomenon. When a phenomenon is ascribed to suggestion we have learnt little more than that it belongs to the sphere of "complex thinking," and is therefore due to the action of an emotional, or more properly, instinctive factor. Such a classification can obviously form only a first stage of the investigation, and to obtain anything that can be reasonably called a complete explanation we must ascertain the particular emotional factor at work, and the precise circumstances

---

[1] *Loc. cit.*

[2] W. Trotter, *Instincts of the Herd in Peace and War*, London, 1915.

[3] Ernest Jones, "The action of Suggestion in Psychotherapy" (*Papers on Psychoanalysis*, 2nd edition, London, 1918).

in which it acts. This criticism applies to many of the attempts that have been made to explain the mechanism of the psychoneuroses, such as the theory of Babinski and his followers which postulates suggestion as the essential cause of hysteria. This theory demonstrates an obvious fact of observation, but leaves out everything worth explaining—why the patient is so abnormally suggestible, what is the particular emotional force responsible for the suggestion, and why he has developed these particular symptoms and not others. The answer that is sometimes given to these further inquiries, that the patient has an hysterical constitution, is a refuge strictly comparable to Molière's famous explanation of the hypnotic properties of opium, but hardly worthy of admission within the portals of science.

Another word frequently cited as a convenient explanation for various phenomena is autosuggestion, and here again usage is so loose and ambiguous that the need for definition and limitation is imperative. One sense in which it is used is, for example, to explain the process by which a patient, who is convinced that his arm is paralysed, actually develops a functional paralysis of the arm. Now the process by which the actual paralysis follows the conviction is probably direct and inevitable, the two stages being little more than different aspects of one and the same fact, but whatever its nature may be it has certainly nothing to do with suggestion. The suggestion lies farther back in the sequence of causes, and is responsible for the acceptance with conviction of the proposition that the arm is paralysed. Once this proposition is so accepted the actual paralysis follows inevitably, but by a mechanism in which suggestion plays no further part. In this sense, therefore, in so far as the word is not definitely misleading it is merely tautological. Another sense in which autosuggestion is employed is to designate those varieties of "complex thinking" in which a direct relation between persons is not involved. That is to say, it designates all "complex thinking" except suggestion in the narrowed meaning we have advocated for that word, and is proffered, for example, as an explanation of our politics, prejudices and so forth. Here again the term would seem to be misleading and redundant. A third sense in which autosuggestion is used is to describe a process whereby one seeks to narrow down one's field of consciousness, and to fill it with a single idea as, for instance, when we endeavour to produce a pseudo-hallucinatory sensation by fixing our attention on a small area of our skin. The process here clearly presents some resemblance to the production of similar phenomena by hypnosis, and in this limited sense the use of the word autosuggestion is probably justifiable[1].

We may sum up the position now reached as follows. All the processes ascribed to suggestion are in reality examples of "complex thinking," and how large a section of "complex thinking" is to be included under suggestion is a matter for purely arbitrary selection and limitation. Probably it would be practically advisable to limit the term to processes of communication involving a direct relation between persons, but even here no specific elements are present. In every case the only essential feature is the action of an emotional or instinctive factor, and this is the essential feature of all "complex thinking." Processes of this kind are, however, so common in the human mind that to explain any particular phenomenon by ascribing it to "complex thinking" or to "suggestion" is altogether inadequate. The explanation can only be accepted as satisfying and complete when we have ascertained the particular emotional factors responsible,

[1] Since the date of this paper a theory and practice of autosuggestion has been developed by Coué and his followers which has attained a great vogue in recent years. Their conception of autosuggestion would seem to belong essentially to the third sense described above. Its relation to suggestion has been considered in detail in Dr Ernest Jones' paper (*loc. cit.*), see also Lecture I.

THE METHODS OF PSYCHOTHERAPY

and the conditions under which they have produced their results.

This preliminary investigation of the nature of suggestion has necessarily been somewhat lengthy, but it has enabled us to achieve a standpoint from which our main problem, the use of suggestion as a therapeutic agent, may be easily attacked. The therapeutic aim of suggestion is to implant in the mind of the patient a certain conviction, and this conviction generally consists in the firm belief that a symptom has disappeared, or is about to disappear. Its utility in the psychoneuroses is dependent on the fact that many of the symptoms of these disorders are the result of beliefs held with conviction by the patient. However intricate and lengthy the chain of causation which has produced them may be, the penultimate link in the chain is the conviction that certain symptoms are present. A functional paralysis of the arm, for example, may be the final result of a long chain of psychical causes, but the penultimate link is the conviction that the arm is paralysed. Now the object of suggestion is to destroy that conviction by implanting in the mind the opposite conviction, namely that the arm is not paralysed, and if this process is successful the chain of causation is broken at its penultimate link, and the symptom disappears. Suggestion is able to accomplish this by virtue of its capacity for inhibiting conflicting ideas and tendencies, whereby the action of the ideas and tendencies responsible for the symptom is blocked, and the conviction communicated by the suggestion is permitted to flourish unchecked. This capacity is dependent upon the employment of an emotional or instinctive factor, and, in the narrower conception of suggestion we have proposed, this emotional or instinctive factor is one involving a direct relation between two persons, the doctor and the patient. The consideration of the wider question, how far and in what way emotional or instinctive factors which do not involve this direct

relation between persons may be employed as therapeutic agents, will be postponed until we have considered
the nature of the second basic principle, persuasion.

PERSUASION

Persuasion, like suggestion, is a term of regrettably
vague and ambiguous character. It is used in the literature in two quite distinct senses, which may be fathered
upon Dubois[1] and Dejerine[2] respectively. For Dubois it
is a purely logical process, for Dejerine it is a logical
process, but one in which affective factors play a necessary
and important part. These two conceptions must naturally be dealt with separately. Dubois conceives persuasion as a process in which certain effects are produced by
chains of logical reasoning, and distinguishes it sharply
from suggestion. The latter is dependent upon blind
faith, while the former appeals to clear logical reason.
Now, if we bear in mind the analysis of the nature of
suggestion which has already been made, the relationship
to it of Dubois's conception of persuasion is immediately
apparent. This relationship is identical with that which
exists between "rational thinking" and "complex
thinking." In the former the stream of consciousness
proceeds in a direction determined entirely by the intrinsic values of its elements, each step being the logical
consequence of the preceding steps. Emotional factors
play no part, and the conclusion follows inevitably from
the premises, just as a proposition of Euclid inevitably
leads us along a road fixed by the logical relationship of
its terms. The conclusion can be predicted with certainty
by an observer who knows only the proposition, and
nothing at all of the man who is thinking it. In "complex
thinking," on the other hand, the direction of the stream

[1] P. Dubois, *The Psychic Treatment of Nervous Disorders*, New
York and London, 1909.
[2] Dejerine and Gauckler, *The Psychoneuroses and their treatment
by Psychotherapy*, English translation, Philad. and London, 1913.

of consciousness is conditioned by emotional factors
which force it into a path which will subserve the aim of
the emotional system in question, and which distort the
logical relationship of its elements so that this aim may
be achieved. Here the conclusion cannot be predicted
unless the observer knows not only the proposition, but
also the man who thinks it and the emotional systems
which dominate his mental activity.

If persuasion is identical with rational thinking then
it is clear that the superiority to suggestion which Dubois
claims for it is based on very solid grounds, for rational
thinking leads to knowledge, whereas suggestion leads
only to beliefs erected upon an insecure foundation. The
sole question which arises is how far rational thinking
can be used for therapeutic ends, and how far it is capable
of destroying the convictions responsible for psychoneurotic symptoms, for the impotence of logic against
the creations of an emotional system is a phenomenon
which is only too frequent and obvious. In practice,
indeed, it will be found that the utility of Dubois's
persuasion is severely limited on account of this
difficulty, but it is nevertheless indubitable that it has
utility.

The therapeutic employment of persuasion is dependent upon a process which in its final stages is identical
with that which occurs in suggestion. We have seen that
many of the symptoms of the psychoneuroses are the
result of beliefs held with conviction by the patient, and
that, however intricate the chain of causation may be,
the penultimate link is the conviction that certain
symptoms are present. Now the aim of persuasion, just
as the aim of suggestion, is to implant in the mind of the
patient the opposite conviction, namely that the symptoms have disappeared, or are about to disappear. This
is explicitly stated by Dubois in the following words:
"The nervous patient is on the path to recovery as soon
as he has the conviction that he is going to be cured; he

is cured on the day when he believes himself to be cured."[1]
To take again the example formerly selected to illustrate
the action of suggestion, that of functional paralysis of
the arm. If this condition is treated by persuasion the
aim, just as before, is to destroy the conviction that the
arm is paralysed, upon which the actual paralysis is
dependent, and to implant in its stead the conviction
that the arm is capable of normal movement. But in this
case the conviction is achieved, not as the effect of an
emotional process, but as the logical result of a chain of
reasoning. It is demonstrated to the patient, for example,
that all the tissues of his arm are healthy, that none of
the signs which inevitably belong to an organic lesion
are present, that the muscles of the arm are actually
capable of work, and so forth. From all these premises
the conclusion that the arm is not paralysed follows as
an inevitable deduction.

Dejerine's conception of persuasion cannot be so easily
described and placed in its relation to other methods.
This difficulty arises, I believe, because his conception
does not correspond to any simple process, but is made
up of a variety of processes essentially different one from
another. In various passages in which he defines persuasion as he understands it, he states, for example, that
persuasion consists in explaining to the patient the true
reasons for his condition, in establishing the patient's
confidence in himself, and in awakening the different
elements of his personality capable of becoming the
starting-point of the effort which will enable him to regain
his self-control; he says, further, that in order that this may
happen an element of feeling must intervene between
the doctor's reasoning and the acceptance of this reasoning
by the patient, and that psychotherapy depends wholly
and exclusively upon the beneficial influence of one
person on another. Now at least three distinct processes
are involved here. Firstly, the explanation to the patient

[1] *Loc. cit.*

of the nature of his condition is a reasoning process identical with the method of Dubois. Secondly, in so far as the effect is dependent upon the beneficial influence of one person on another, it is dependent upon an emotional relation existing between the two persons, and is therefore clearly due to suggestion in the narrower sense. Thirdly, the employment of the various elements of the patient's personality as weapons for achieving the therapeutic end consists essentially in making use of those emotional forces in the patient which do not necessarily involve a direct emotional relation to the doctor, and is therefore identical with "complex thinking" in general. This third process is the only one which we have not already investigated. It will be remembered that, at the end of the section on suggestion, we postponed for later consideration the question how far and in what way emotional or instinctive factors which do not involve a direct relation between persons may be employed as therapeutic agents. This question must now be examined, for it is evident that the third process contained in Dejerine's method is an attempt to provide a practical answer to it.

We have seen that most of the movements of our mental machinery are due to the driving power exerted by emotional systems, that these systems direct the stream of consciousness into channels which will subserve their goal, and that a great part of our beliefs and opinions are due to agencies of this character. Now it is clear that, by suitable stimulation and combination of the emotional systems existing in our patients, effects can be obtained which will have a therapeutic value. Thus, by making use of the religion, ambitions, affections and other weapons which are available in the patient's mind, we may be able to destroy or mould into other forms the mental processes responsible for his symptoms. The effect here is due to the employment of emotional factors, but it is not mainly due to the employment of an emotional relation existing between the doctor and the patient. It is in other words the result of "complex thinking," but not the result of suggestion in the narrow sense. The part played by the doctor here is comparable to the action of an engine driver, who merely directs the forces produced in the engine.

This process constitutes one of the most powerful and efficient weapons in our therapeutic armoury, and we shall subsequently see that it is employed, to some extent at least, by all psychotherapists, to whatever school they may profess to belong. Sometimes it is used merely as a method of removing symptoms, the object being, just as in the case of suggestion, to produce in the patient a conviction that the symptoms have disappeared or are about to disappear. In other cases, however, it is used as a means of readjusting the causes which are ultimately responsible for the symptoms. Here the previous elucidation of the causes by some analytical method is necessarily presupposed, and we may now pass on to investigate the nature of these analytical methods.

ANALYTICAL METHODS

The term "analysis" is used in this paper to indicate any method whereby the nature and relationship of the causes responsible for the patient's condition are determined, and the condition removed by the rearrangement and readjustment of these causes. It is not meant to be synonymous with psychoanalysis, a word which should only be applied to the method devised by Freud and generally associated with his name. Psychoanalysis is clearly analysis, but the latter is a wider term and one applicable to all therapeutic procedures which satisfy the definition given above. It is unquestionable, of course, that all modern analytical methods owe a great debt to the work of Freud, and that in each and every one of them many of his essential principles are incor-

porated. Psychoanalysis, however, involves the acceptance of a particular theory of causation, and should not
be used to designate methods which are not governed by
this theory.

The employment of analysis as a therapeutic measure
is based on the assumption that certain disorders are of
psychogenic origin. If this assumption is admitted, if it
is agreed that some disorders are the result of a chain
of mental causes, then it is immediately obvious that
treatment should aim at elucidating those causes, and
then so altering or rearranging them that their original
effect is no longer produced. This procedure is so evidently demanded by all the canons of scientific medicine
that the point is hardly worth labouring.

How many and what disorders are to be included in
the psychogenic group is a question which cannot be
fully answered in the present state of our knowledge.
We are yet uncertain, for example, how far the various
types of insanity can be brought under this head. So far
as the psychoneuroses are concerned, however, the view
that they are essentially of psychogenic origin has steadily
gained ground during the past fifty years, and has been
so confirmed and extended by the experiences of the War,
that it would be fair to say that it is now accepted by
almost every authority in every country. If this is so,
then clearly the analytical method of treatment is
eminently applicable to these disorders. Dispute can
only arise as to the nature and action of the causes responsible, and the relative merits of different methods
of ascertaining and removing them. It is upon differences
of opinion with regard to these matters that the divergent
therapeutic procedures adopted by various authorities are
based, but the examination and criticism of these differences would take us far beyond the limits of this paper,
which aims only at the consideration of broad general
principles.

RELATION OF SUGGESTION, PERSUASION, AND ANALYSIS AS THERAPEUTIC METHODS

We are now in a position to consider the relation between suggestion, persuasion, and analysis as therapeutic methods. Analysis is distinguished from the other two in that it is aimed at the causes responsible for the condition, and seeks to remove the condition by removing

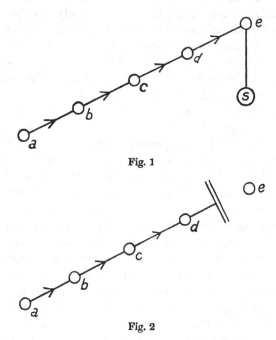

Fig. 1

Fig. 2

or rearranging those causes, whereas suggestion and persuasion, in so far as they are not combined with analysis, are aimed solely at the symptom, and seek to remove the symptoms without reference to the causes which have produced them. This distinction may be made clear with the aid of the above diagrams.

Fig. 1 represents the chain of causation responsible for the appearance of certain symptoms, a, b, c, d, e;

indicate causal factors, and s the symptoms produced
by their interaction[1]. In a large number of the symptoms
of the psychoneuroses the penultimate link (e) will consist in the conviction that a certain symptom is present,
and from this penultimate link the symptom itself follows
directly in the manner already described. Now if this
condition is treated by suggestion, attention is directed
solely to the penultimate link, and an endeavour is made
to destroy this, and to substitute for it the conviction
that the symptom is not present (e^1). If the procedure is
successful the symptom promptly disappears, because
the chain of causation responsible for it is broken. The
break is effected, however, only at the penultimate link;
the causes, a, b, c, d, are left *in situ*, and the situation
achieved is as represented in Fig. 2. It will be clear that,
as the primary causes have not been attacked, there is
an obvious possibility either of relapse or of the development of another similar symptom, a possibility noto-
riously borne out by clinical experience.

If, next, the symptom is treated by pure persuasion, a
very similar state of affairs is produced. The aim as
before is to destroy the penultimate link (e), and to substitute for it the conviction that the symptom is not
present. This is accomplished here, however, not by
implanting the conviction with the aid of an emotional
factor, but by collecting together trains of thought which
will lead to the conviction by their intrinsic logical force.
The situation now is represented by Fig. 3, where f, g
and h indicate the trains of thought in question which
have produced the conviction (e^1) that the symptom is
not present. The symptom disappears just as in the case
of treatment by suggestion, and for the same reason; it
will be observed, moreover, that the primary causes are

---

[1] The diagram is, of course, purely schematic and unduly
simplistic. The causes would be represented more properly by a
network of circles than a line of circles, but this has been omitted
in order to avoid complicating the figure.

again left untouched. This similarity between the two
methods of treatment is evidently not always appreciated
by the exponents of pure persuasion, for it indicates that
the vaunted superiority of persuasion is of doubtful
validity. It may be said, however, that it is unquestionably superior to suggestion in that the removal of the
symptom is achieved by an integrating process presumably more stable than the mere implantation of a belief
without support or foundation.

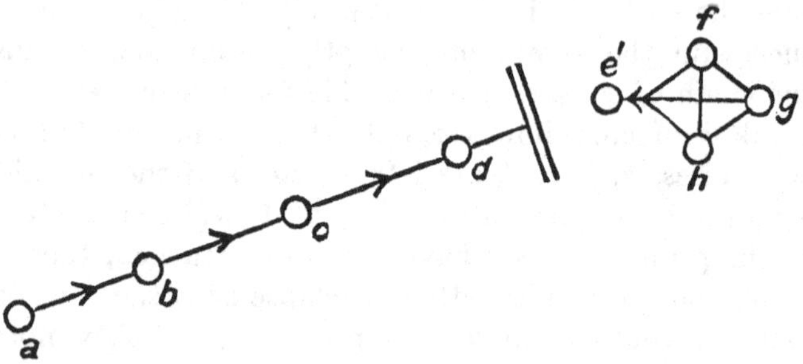

Fig. 3

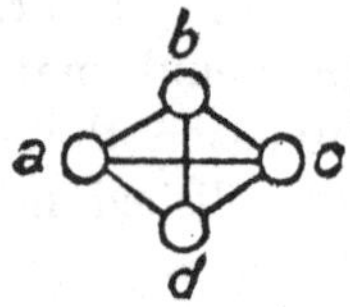

Fig. 4

If, lastly, the symptom is treated by analysis, attention
is directed, not merely to the penultimate link, but to
all the links in the chain of causation. When these have
been ascertained an endeavour is made to destroy or to
rearrange them in such a manner that they are no longer
capable of producing their original effect, namely the
symptom. If this is successful the symptom again disappears, but it disappears now because the whole chain
of causation has been fundamentally altered. The situation thus attained is represented by Fig. 4, where a, b, c

and d have been rearranged in a new pattern which no longer leads to e or s.

The processes crudely illustrated by these diagrams will be rendered more comprehensible by the consideration of an hypothetical case. We will suppose that we are required to treat an hysterical monoplegia of the right arm occurring in a soldier who has been buried by a shell explosion. This symptom is not the result of a single cause, but of a concatenation of causes, amongst which the following may all have played a part. The patient sustained a trifling injury to his arm in childhood, which did not produce any noteworthy physical effect, but made a lasting impression on his mind. Secondly, he had been assured by his relatives, and possibly by his doctor, that as a result of the injury the right arm would always be weaker than the left. Thirdly, when the shell burst a sandbag fell on the right arm. Fourthly, the soldier had been suffering for some time previous to the final shell explosion from a gradually increasing "nervousness" and anxiety, due to the conflict between the opposing forces of self-preservation and discipline, the conflict which is the characteristic feature of the war neuroses. This conflict had latterly become acute, and it was a biological necessity that some solution of the situation should occur. Hence had arisen the unconscious motive which is an integral factor in the causation of all psychoneuroses, the motive which desires a disability as the only solution whereby the conflict can be satisfactorily relieved. As a result of the interaction of all these, and perhaps of other causes, the penultimate link (e), the conviction that the arm was paralysed, was produced, and the actual paralysis followed inevitably.

Now, if this condition is treated by suggestion, our object is to produce the conviction that the arm is not paralysed. This is achieved by hypnosis or other method of suggestion, and the paralysis promptly disappears. No attention whatever is paid to the causes which produced the symptom. Their original outlet is blocked, but they are left as a pathogenic focus whence may develop similar or other symptoms. If, on the other hand, the condition is treated by persuasion, we seek to prove to the patient by a logical demonstration that his arm is not paralysed. We show him that all the tissues are healthy, that the signs which should accompany a real paralysis are absent, that if we lift his arm and then remove the support while his attention is diverted the arm does not drop immediately, and that therefore his muscles must actually be functioning. By collecting together these and similar arguments we shake and finally destroy the conviction on which the paralysis is dependent, and when this aim has been attained the paralysis inevitably disappears. But it will be observed that here again the causes primarily responsible for the paralysis have not been investigated or attacked, and the pathogenic focus is left untouched, just as in the case of suggestion. If, finally, the condition is treated by analysis, all the causes mentioned above are first unearthed, and then an attempt is made to destroy or rearrange them. This latter process may consist, for example, in bringing the various factors into the full light of consciousness, making their relationship and significance apparent to the patient, and subjecting them to the solvent action of the forces available in the patient's mind, his ambitions, self-respect, religion, traditions, or whatever other weapon can be pressed into service. It will be clear that we are employing here the process which was found to form a part of Dejerine's conception of persuasion, the utilising of the emotional factors existing in the patient's mind as weapons capable of readjusting and integrating the mental elements responsible for the symptoms. But in this case the method is applied to the causes ultimately responsible, which have been elucidated by analysis, and not merely to the symptoms themselves.

These considerations lead to the conclusion that analysis

is obviously superior to the other methods we have considered, and it might be supposed that it ought always to be used to the exclusion of the others. This would be an erroneous deduction, however, because it is found in practice that a considerable number of conditions can be dealt with more rapidly and conveniently by the employment of suggestion or persuasion. Certain hysterical symptoms, such, for example, as paralysis, functional gaits, mutism and so forth, can be removed with ease and speed by suggestion or persuasion, which would involve a lengthy and complicated procedure were they treated solely by analysis. It may be said, nevertheless, that even in these cases treatment is far from being adequate and complete unless the removal of the prominent symptoms is followed by an analysis aimed at the elucidation and rearrangement of the ultimate causes. Only in this way can a reasonable stability and freedom from relapse be secured. Cases where the mere employment of suggestion or persuasion has produced apparently solid cures are frequent enough, but this is probably due to the fact that an alteration of the primary causes has been effected by some means independent of the actual treatment. A war hysteric, for example, may have his symptoms removed by suggestion, and may then be discharged from the army, so that the most important of the ultimate causes, the conflict between self-preservation and duty, is rendered inert. Reasons of this kind no doubt help to explain the fact that treatment by suggestion or persuasion is often far more efficient and satisfactory in war psychoneuroses than in the psychoneuroses of the civilian. In any case the sphere of these methods is certainly limited, and they are only capable of application to a comparatively small section of the great group of the psychoneuroses. It would seem, indeed, that they are applicable only to those cases in which the penultimate link in the chain of causation consists in the conviction that a certain symptom is present. Where this link is absent, and where psychical causes have produced symptoms without its intervention, suggestion and persuasion by themselves seem to be impotent. This holds for example in the anxiety neuroses, which bulk largely amongst the war cases, and in which analytical methods of one kind or another are a necessity.

Throughout this paper suggestion, persuasion, and analysis have been sharply distinguished from one another, and regarded as independent methods of treatment. This has been necessary for the purpose of investigating and correlating the basic principles involved. It has already been indicated, however, that in actual practice no school of thought relies exclusively on any one of the three, and that every psychotherapist employs at least two and often all three principles. The practitioner who confines himself to suggestion is impotent when faced with many types of psychoneuroses, and crude and inadequate in his treatment of all types. Dubois employs a certain amount of analysis, and a considerable dose of suggestion. A perusal of Dejerine's work provides instance after instance of the use of analysis, and the employment of affective factors is an integral part of his method. Some of these affective factors clearly belong to suggestion, however narrowly we may define that term, and all of them come under that general conception of "complex thinking," which is identified with suggestion by many authorities, and is most certainly closely allied thereto. A similar criticism applies to all the analytical schools. If it be agreed, indeed, that the driving forces of the mind are all ultimately dependent upon the interplay of instincts, then it is clear that without these emotional factors the mind cannot do anything, and nothing can be done to the mind.

CONCLUSION

We may now attempt to sum up the conclusions reached in the foregoing pages. It was originally stated

that all methods of psychotherapy are dependent upon
the employment of one or more of three basic principles,
suggestion, persuasion, and analysis. Our investigation
has shown, however, that suggestion is a term of vague
and indefinite connotation, ranging in meaning from a
conception identical with "complex thinking" to a conception covering only the phenomena observed in
hypnosis, and closely allied phenomena. Under these
circumstances it would seem advisable to employ some
other term to indicate that wider conception of suggestion
which includes within its boundaries any employment
of affective factors as curative agents, and to limit
suggestion to those instances where the affective factors
are those involving a direct relation between the doctor
and the patient. A wider term which would seem appropriate for this purpose is "affective therapeutics." Our
original statement would then be modified so as to read
that all methods of psychotherapy are dependent upon
the employment of one or more of three basic principles,
affective therapeutics, persuasion, and analysis. The
characters of these three principles may be described as
follows.

Affective therapeutics consists in the employment of
the various emotional, or more properly instinctive,
factors existing in the patient's mind, as weapons whereby
pathogenic mental processes may be destroyed or altered.
The method is dependent upon the property possessed
by these emotional factors of furthering tendencies in
harmony with them and inhibiting opposing tendencies.
When the emotional factor employed consists in an
affective relationship between doctor and patient the
process becomes suggestion in the narrow sense. When
the factors employed do not involve this direct relationship, then we have the process which is an integral part
of Dejerine's persuasion, as it is indeed of all psychotherapeutic methods, but which is clearly distinct from
the persuasion of Dubois.

Persuasion, in the sense of Dubois, consists in an endeavour to destroy a pathogenic mental process by reasoning, the effect being produced not by any emotional factor but by the logical force of the arguments presented to the patient. In itself this method is probably almost impotent, but combined with affective therapeutics it becomes a powerful and efficient weapon.

Analysis consists in an investigation of the causes responsible for the patient's condition, and the removal of the condition by the removal or alteration of the causes.

These three principles can be clearly distinguished theoretically, but in actual practice more than one principle is almost inevitably employed. Every psychotherapist, although he may style himself suggestionist, persuasionist, or analyst, makes use of at least two and often of all three principles. Suggestion and persuasion by themselves have but a limited field of application; they are only capable of dealing with symptoms, and probably only with symptoms which are directly dependent upon the existence in the patient's mind of a certain conviction. Affective therapeutics, other than suggestion in the narrow sense, has a wider application, but its use as an accurate weapon pre-supposes a preliminary analysis. Analysis is clearly the ideal method, but it is more properly a stage in treatment rather than a method complete in itself. By its employment the various causal factors responsible for the disordered condition are elucidated, but when this has been achieved there remains the further task of rearranging or eliminating these causal factors, and in this latter process persuasion and affective therapeutics are probably invariably called into play.

Practical psychotherapy, therefore, necessarily involves an admixture of principles, and this admixture will be there however the physician may endeavour to exclude it. Suggestion, for example, is omnipresent, and will obviously come into action wherever there is a doctor and a patient. It is surely better then that this action should be correctly estimated and deliberately utilised rather than left to the vagaries of chance. The task of the physician is to cure the patient, and in order to achieve this end he should be prepared to make use of any and every weapon which lies to his hand. Affective therapeutics, persuasion, and analysis all have their place, but treatment can only be efficient if their nature and limitations are clearly understood, so that the physician may choose and combine his weapons according to the condition which has to be attacked.

THE CONCEPTION OF DISSOCIATION[1]

DISSOCIATION, in the sense in which it is understood
in modern psychology, was first fashioned into a clearly
defined conception by the work of Janet. The general
notion of a division in the mind, however, has a far more
remote ancestry. It may be said, indeed, that the whole
history of psychology consists in the enumeration of successive attempts to carve discrete parts out of that con-
tinuum which we call mind. These attempts are apparent,
for example, in the dissection by the academic psychologist of subjective experience into sensations, perceptions,
emotions, conations and so forth, in the mosaic picture
of mind created by the associationists, in the various
classifications of mental processes into conscious, subconscious and unconscious, which take us by way of Janet
to the earlier conceptions of Freud, and finally in the
demarcation of ego and id which marks Freud's later
work. The divisions enumerated are not all made on the
same plane. This difference of plane is obvious enough
when we compare the dissection of mind into perceptions,
emotions, and conations, with its dissection into ego and
id, but it is not so obvious when we compare the latter
with the type of division established by Janet in his conception of dissociation. Nevertheless the difference of
plane exists as much here, and is as important in its
significance and consequences. The aim of the present
paper is to consider the nature of Janet's conceptions of
dissociation and of the subconscious, to elucidate the
difference of plane which marks off these conceptions

[1] A Presidential Address to the Medical Section of the British
Psychological Society, December 15th, 1926, and subsequently
published in the *British Journal of Medical Psychology*, vol. vi,
part 1, 1926.

from those created by Freud, and to discuss the relationships and oppositions which exist between them.

The hypothesis that mental elements may exist outside the limits of ordinary consciousness can be traced far back in the history of philosophy. In one of its forms these extra-conscious elements, e.g. the "petites perceptions" of Leibniz, were regarded as being identical in nature with the constituents of normal consciousness, and differing from the latter only in intensity. This corresponds to the "fringe of consciousness" of later psychologists, and describes a range of phenomena which has nothing to do with the conceptions we are now examining, although the term "subconscious" is sometimes confusingly applied thereto. In another of its forms, however, the hypothesis assumes that mental processes exist outside consciousness, which are radically different from those occurring within consciousness, but which are able to modify and affect the course of the latter. This notion is to be found in Kant and Schopenhauer, and is elaborately developed in Hartmann's *Philosophy of the Unconscious*. It is clearly to be regarded as the logical ancestor of the Freudian "unconscious."

Janet's conception of dissociation, however, developed along an entirely different line[1]. It was not a conception which was designed, or could be applied, to explain mental processes in general, but was formulated to explain, or rather to describe, a limited class of phenomena, in particular those met with in hysteria and hypnosis. Janet observed in these conditions definite evidence that mental elements and processes could preserve an independent existence apart from the main stream of consciousness. He showed, for example, that the sensations arising from the anaesthetic limb of an hysterical patient had not been destroyed, but were merely cut off from the central consciousness. Their continued existence could not only be inferred from certain facts in the patient's behaviour, such

[1] Cf. pp. 35 ff.

as the remarkable freedom from accidental injury enjoyed by the anaesthetic limb, but directly demonstrated by procedures which enabled the dissociated stream of consciousness to be tapped, hypnosis and automatic writing for instance. A similar explanation could be applied to the amnesias of hysteria. Somnambulisms, again, were the result of a dissociation which cut across the stream of consciousness, and permitted the stage to be occupied by a new stream having no apparent link with that which had preceded it. Moreover, this new stream contained memories and themes of which the normal consciousness had no knowledge, but whose continued existence during periods when no somnambulism was in progress could be shown by hypnosis or automatic writing. Fugues and double personalities were clearly more complicated examples of the same mechanism, and finally Janet concluded that all the phenomena of hysteria were to be regarded as instances of dissociation, a dissociation in which he saw the essential feature of the disorder. As dissociation of the same type was evidently a character of hypnosis, Janet naturally followed Charcot's lead, and held that hypnosis was an artificial hysteria.

The value of Janet's conception as a weapon of understanding is beyond question, and it has cast a flood of light upon some of the problems of hypnosis and hysteria. Nevertheless it presents certain defects and inconsistencies which, at any rate in the form in which Janet cast it, oppose considerable difficulties in the way of its complete acceptance. Janet is a descendant of the associationists, and he talks glibly of the sticking together and unsticking of bits of mind-stuff, in a manner which is repugnant to the psychology of to-day. Moreover, his conception of dissociation is constructed in that spatial metaphor which so often produces a superficial appearance of clarity at the expense of a gross distortion of the underlying facts. Dissociation is for Janet the separation *en masse* of a number of mental elements from that greater aggregation of elements which constitutes the totality of the mind, a splitting of the mind into two independent pieces. Now this picture cannot be satisfactorily reconciled with the observed facts. To begin with, the same material may form part of each of the dissociated portions. Each of two dissociated personalities, for example, may possess the same memories. The existence of such common elements does not seem to be compatible with the notion of dissociation as a separation of two masses of mental atoms. Again, Dr T. W. Mitchell[1] has pointed out that the relationships of awareness and lack of awareness existing between the separate streams of consciousness do not show that simple character which the notion of a spatial dissociation would require. An hypnotic consciousness may be aware of the whole range of the patient's experience, including the content of the normal consciousness, while the normal consciousness has no knowledge whatever of the experience belonging to the hypnotic consciousness. The dissociation here, instead of producing a barrier equally untraversable in either direction, shows itself in one direction only, the content of the normal consciousness being perfectly accessible to the hypnotic, while an impassable gap is interposed whenever we endeavour to move in the reverse way. Dr Mitchell has further objected to Janet's notion of a dissociated idea existing in a wholly isolated state. "It cannot be too often repeated and insisted on that we have absolutely no knowledge of any such isolated mental material. If normally an experience that passes out of consciousness is conserved as a psychical disposition, it is as a psychical disposition which is part of *some* personality....Its dissociated status has reference to the supraliminal consciousness and to that alone. It is not cut off on all sides from the structure of the mind, but only deprived of those associative connexions which would permit its emergence above the

[1] T. W. Mitchell, *The Psychology of Medicine*, London, 1921, p. 33.

threshold. It is dissociated from the supraliminal consciousness, but is still an integral part of the mind beneath the threshold[1]."

Similar difficulties arise when we endeavour to apply this conception of a splitting of mental elements from a larger aggregate, to the phenomena of trance personalities. Here nothing is apparently removed from the normal consciousness, and the content of the secondary consciousness seems to have a quite independent development. In Sidis' well-known Hanna case, again, the dissociated personality appeared to be at first without content, consisting in nothing but a bare consciousness, a blank form which only gradually became filled in. Here the conception of a segregated mass of mental elements is clearly inadequate. It fails also when applied to cases of coconscious double personality, the cases where there is not merely an alternation of personalities, but a contemporaneous co-existence of two personalities, one of which is aware of, but nevertheless entirely independent of, the mental activity of the other. Sally in the Beauchamp case, for example, not only occasionally occupied the stage as an alternating personality, but appeared to persist as a coconscious personality when other personalities were on the stage, aware of and therefore in some sense connected with these other personalities, but preserving her own individuality. Here there is a complex inter-relationship of the dissociated systems, which cannot be clearly represented by any conception couched in a spatial metaphor. An analogous complex inter-relationship is well illustrated by certain phenomena observed in a case of double personality which was under my care some sixteen years ago[2]. I propose to interrupt the thread of my argument for a moment in order to describe the broad features of

[1] T. W. Mitchell, *Medical Psychology and Psychical Research*, London, 1922, p. 113.

[2] Bernard Hart, "A case of double personality," *Journal of Mental Science*, 1912.

this case, because it serves to illustrate not only the points now under discussion, but also others which will be dealt with later.

The patient, whom we will call John Smith, was admitted to a mental hospital with a history of fugues occurring at intervals throughout some years. During each fugue he wandered about the country, behaving in a more or less irresponsible manner, and on the last occasion exhibiting abnormalities of conduct which led to his certification. At the termination of each fugue he returned suddenly to his normal condition, with a total amnesia for everything that had happened since the onset of the fugue. At the time of his admission to the hospital, therefore, the history which he was able to give of his recent life was marked by a series of blanks, the blanks extending over varying periods from a few days to several weeks.

The lost memories were recovered by the use of hypnosis, and an attempt was then made to push the investigation further, and to discover the factors responsible for the fugues. It was during this process of further investigation that the second personality made its appearance. I was at the time questioning him about a remarkable dislike which he evinced towards one of his relatives. The patient's demeanour, which had hitherto always been very courteous, rapidly changed. He burst into a rage, and when I mentioned certain facts he had previously communicated to me, denied that he had ever said any such things. He asserted that he had only seen me once before, and laughed contemptuously when I pointed out that we had had at least twenty prolonged interviews. After a few minutes he suddenly sat down, complained of headache, and in a few seconds returned to his usual condition, with a complete amnesia for the whole period that the second personality had been on the stage.

After this episode the new personality frequently appeared, and I christened it the "one-fifth man," the name originating from a conversation with the patient in which I explained to him that sometimes four-fifths of him was on the stage, sometimes one-fifth.

The one-fifth man underwent a rapid development, and was subsequently a much more complicated person than on the occasion of his first appearance. He was always, however, suspicious and hostile, and with an unconcealed aversion to myself. He was, moreover, always blankly ignorant of all the material previously recovered in the investigation, and angrily incredulous whenever these subjects were touched upon. He had a perfect memory for his own former appearances, but none for the periods when the four-fifths personality held the field. The latter, by the way, was always courteous, friendly, grateful for the trouble I was taking over his case, and distressed when I showed him the abusive letters which the one-fifth man frequently sent to me. It should be noted that the secondary personality was in no way identical with the fugues which occurred before the patient's admission, and had no knowledge whatever of the events of the fugue periods.

Experience soon showed that the one-fifth man was always produced by any attempt to push the investigation in certain directions, and I was able to bring him on to the stage whenever I liked by deliberately employing this procedure. The one-fifth man could, indeed, be regarded as a kind of crystallized resistance.

The one-fifth man preserved his attributes as a resistance throughout his entire career, but the hostility to me did not permanently persist. Hostility to an individual remained a constant character, but it was occasionally transferred to some individual other than myself. It was transferred, for example, during one considerable period on to a certain official of the hospital. In this phase the one-fifth man bitterly reviled this official as a maligner and a spy, but he was then entirely friendly to me.

An episode, which occurred on the first occasion when an attempt was made to control the activities of the one-fifth man, affords an excellent illustration of the impossibility of conceiving adequately the dissociations in this case in any kind of spatial terminology. When it appeared likely that the hostile character of the one-fifth man might lead to awkward complications, a suggestion was given during hypnosis to the effect that, if a certain small metal object were exhibited on any occasion when the one-fifth man happened to be present, then the ordinary personality would immediately return. Some time afterwards, in the course of a difficult interview with the one-fifth man, I decided to try the effectiveness of the suggestion which had been given. The patient at the moment had his back to me, and was gazing out of the window pursuing his customary occupation of reviling myself and all my works. I requested him to "turn round and look at this." To my astonishment he absolutely refused to do anything of the sort, resolutely kept his back to me, and it was only by the exertion of some physical force that he was finally constrained to look at the metal object. Directly he did so the ordinary personality reappeared, with his usual complete amnesia for everything which had happened since the advent of the one-fifth man. On various later occasions the one-fifth man displayed incredible ingenuity in a systematic campaign to obtain possession of the metal object, even going so far as to attempt to bribe the servants to procure it for him. When I asked him what he would do if he succeeded, he replied that he would stand with his back to the drawer in which he believed it to be kept, drop it behind him, and stamp on it. In this way he thought he would be able to free himself from my interference in his affairs.

In order to appreciate the significance of these facts it is necessary to remember that neither the ordinary personality nor the one-fifth man were aware of the content of the hypnotic consciousness, or of the post-hypnotic suggestion which had been given. Yet the reluctance of the one-fifth man to turn round can only have been due to some kind of knowledge on his part that the action would be lethal to him. For it is to be noted that the situation is not comparable to that present in an ordinary post-hypnotic suggestion, where the suggestion is carried out, possibly with the knowledge of, but without any interference from, the normal consciousness. The action of the one-fifth man must have been dictated by an appreciation and understanding of the significance of the post-hypnotic suggestion, and of the result which it would produce, this appreciation and understanding being entirely unconscious, and only manifesting themselves in consciousness as a blind resistance to carrying out the order. The resistance cannot be ascribed to a learning by previous experience of the lethal power of the metal object, because the resistance appeared on the first occasion on which the object was so employed. Now the spatial conception of dissociation permits us to attribute the action to the one-fifth personality, and the suggestion to the hypnotic consciousness, but there is no place for the appreciation and understanding which mediate between the two and yet belong to neither.

An analogous situation exists in the well-known "Yes and No" test for hysterical anaesthesia, where the patient answers "Yes" when touched on the sound limb and "No" when touched on the anaesthetic limb. Here, again, the answering of "No" indicates the mediation of an unconscious appreciation and understanding between the dissociated consciousness which is aware of the sensation, and the normal consciousness which ignores it. Both in this instance and in the episode of the one-fifth man we seem to require something beyond the two dissociated streams of consciousness in order to explain the facts, a consideration which points, as we shall see later, in the direction of the Freudian "unconscious."

Some of the difficulties in the application of the conception of dissociation disappear if we abandon the atomistic and spatial terminology in which the conception was originally described. Naturally the phenomena with which we are concerned are in reality absolutely devoid of any actual spatial aspect, and the introduction of a spatial metaphor, although it lends itself insidiously to the construction of attractive diagrams, can only lead to erroneous deductions unless its purely descriptive and illustrative function is rigidly controlled. Dissociation does not separate the mind into pieces, it only produces more or less independently acting functional units, each such unit comprising material which may be peculiar to itself, but which may just as well form a part of any number of other functional units. The distinguishing character does not lie in the material of which it is composed, but in the set or pattern. Instead of regarding dissociation as the splitting of conscious material into separate masses, it must be regarded as an affair of gearing, the various elements of mental machinery being organised into different functional systems by the throwing in of the appropriate gear, or, if it is desired to render the situation in physiological terms, we have the notion of engrams and neuronic patterns developed in Dr R. G. Gordon's recent book[1]. With this conception the difficulty in understanding how the same material can belong to several personalities, or how there can be a non-reciprocal amnesia between the normal and hypnotic consciousness, is largely overcome.

The spatial and functional conceptions of dissociation are radically distinct from one another in their angle of approach to the phenomena which they seek to describe. The former regards the dissociated consciousness as built up by the accretion of elements, the simplest example being provided by the cases where only a few such elements are dissociated, hysterical anaesthesia for instance, while the more complex cases are produced by the addition of more and more elements to the dissociated mass, until finally that mass attains dimensions to which the term "personality" may reasonably be ascribed. The functional conception, on the contrary, starts at the other end. It lays stress on the synthesising activity which brings the elements together, and regards this as the essential feature rather than the mere agglomeration of elements. Instead of seeing in personality the final result of an unusually extensive agglomeration, it assumes that some synthesising agent comparable to personality is present in every case.

With a functional interpretation of this type the conception of dissociation can be considerably extended,

[1] R. G. Gordon, *Personality*, London, 1926.

and applied to phenomena which could not be subsumed under the spatial interpretation. Several cases of multiple personality have been described in which the different personalities share the same memories, but are sharply distinguished from one another by the diversity of their characters and activities. There seems to be no ground for excluding these cases from the group of multiple personality, although there is no mutual amnesia. Similar considerations apply to those fugues where there is no subsequent amnesia, but where the behaviour during the fugue is totally foreign to that characterising the normal self. Perhaps it is even justifiable to extend the conception to the changes observed in cyclothymia and the manic-depressive psychosis. It can be applied, again, to the interpretation of hallucinations, to those conditions where elaborate delusional systems exist without effect upon the behaviour of the patient, and even to the logic-tight compartment mechanisms observed in everyday life. The objection to this kind of extension is that a generalisation which is stretched over a wide and graded series of phenomena tends to lose its precision and definition, and therefore its utility. It has some value, however, in that it connotes a common factor, i.e. a lack of integration, throughout the whole series, though varying in degree from minor examples up to the complete splits of double personality. It should be noted, by the way, that the extension of the conception of dissociation whereby Janet endeavours to explain the phenomena of psychasthenia, is not an extension of the same order, but a further development of the atomistic notion of dissociation.

It was pointed out at the commencement of this address that the history of psychology shows numerous attempts to establish lines of division in the continuity of the mind. Now the divisions which have so far been considered, the divisions included under dissociation, even in the extended sense of dissociation described above, are divisions of consciousness. The evidence for the existence of a dissociated stream of consciousness is of precisely the same order as that which establishes the existence of any kind of consciousness in people other than ourselves. The dissociated stream is made of the same stuff as the remainder of consciousness, and its peculiarity lies simply in the fact that there is a lack of complete integration between it and the remainder of consciousness. Janet's "subconscious" comprises those instances of dissociation where the lack of integration is such that there is a lack of mutual awareness between the two streams, but in every other respect the processes concerned have all the attributes of consciousness. The division of dissociation is therefore a division within consciousness or, as will be explained later, it is a division on the phenomenal plane.

Now the division created by Freud in his conception of the "unconscious" is a division along an entirely different plane. It is true that the actual history of its development was by way of clinical investigations of much the same kind as those which led to Janet's conception, but, as has already been mentioned, its logical ancestry is altogether different. This ancestry is to be found in the hypotheses which assumed the existence of mental processes lying altogether outside consciousness, but whose activity explained the facts of consciousness, hypotheses formulated by Kant, Schopenhauer, and Hartmann. The unconscious of Freud has been created by him in order to explain the processes occurring in consciousness. It is not in itself a fact of consciousness, and its existence cannot be demonstrated in the way in which the existence of Janet's dissociated streams can be demonstrated, any more than we can demonstrate the existence of the ether which has been created in order to explain the facts of light and heat.

In a paper published in 1909 I endeavoured to formulate and analyse the essential difference of plane existing between the conceptions of Janet and Freud, and the chief conclusions reached therein still seem to me to be fundamentally sound[1]. The "subconscious" of Janet is a description of phenomenal facts, while the "unconscious" of Freud is a conceptual construction, an imagined entity created in order to explain phenomenal facts. The distinction is that which marks, in all branches of science, the difference between a generalisation from observed facts, e.g. the laws of refraction of various coloured lights, and a conceptual construction designed to explain the facts, e.g. the ether and its waves. The validity of a generalisation from observed facts is established by a procedure entirely different from that needed to establish the validity of a conceptual construction. In the former case only observation and experiment are required; the generalisation states that certain phenomena occur under certain conditions, and the demonstration that the phenomena do so occur establishes the generalisation. The conceptual construction, on the other hand, cannot be demonstrated in this way, because the elements of which it is manufactured have no existence on the phenomenal plane. The procedure here is to deduce the consequences which would follow from the conceptual construction, as it is conceived to be and to act, and then to compare these deduced consequences with the phenomena which are actually observed. If the deduced consequences are identical with the observed phenomena, then the validity of the conceptual construction is established.

These considerations lead to the conclusion that the difference of plane between Janet's "subconscious" and Freud's "unconscious" is that which lies between observable phenomena and conceptual constructions. This, indeed, was the conclusion reached in the paper to which I have referred, but there are certain difficulties in the

[1] Bernard Hart, "The Conception of the Subconscious," *Journ. of Abnorm. Psychol.* 1909. Reprinted in Morton Prince's *Subconscious Phenomena*, Boston, 1915. A summary of this paper has been included in the present volume as an appendix to the second Coulstonian Lecture, *vide* pp. 57 ff.

way of its acceptance. It may be objected that the so-called phenomena of psychology, or at any rate of psycho-pathology, are not observed phenomena at all, but inferences. The conscious processes of others cannot be directly observed; they can only be inferred, and such inferences are of the order of conceptual constructions rather than phenomena. If this be so, no rigid line of demarcation can be established in psychology between phenomena and conceptual constructions, and the distinction becomes one of degree rather than of an essential difference in kind. Even if this be admitted, however, the difference of degree between Janet's and Freud's conception is so pronounced as to constitute a fundamental distinction of method, and it is from the side of methodology that the divergence in plane can be best represented. From this standpoint the conscious processes of others, although strictly inferences rather than actually observed phenomena, are treated as observed phenomena.

Karl Pearson[1] has shown that the method of science consists in three steps, firstly the observing and recording of phenomena, secondly the classification of the phenomena observed, and thirdly the construction of formulae or laws which will resume or explain the phenomena[2]. In this third step it is legitimate to use a conceptual imagery, and to construct hypothetical entities conceived to behave in a certain manner. Now if we apply this methodological standard to the conceptions of the subconscious and the unconscious, it is obvious that Janet's dissociation belongs to the second step; it is a classification of observed phenomena, while Freud's unconscious belongs to the third step; it is a conceptual construction. This distinction of plane between subconscious and unconscious, manifesting itself in the radically divergent methods by which the conceptions are reached and by which they can be tested, is of fundamental importance.

[1] Karl Pearson, *The Grammar of Science*, 1892.
[2] Cf. pp. 3 ff.

Unless it is recognised, confusion of thought is inevitable, and it is not difficult to find examples of such confusion. Hitschmann[1], for instance, after quite correctly pointing out that "unconscious, in the Freudian sense,...means something which one does not really know, while one is compelled in the analysis by conclusive inferences to recognize it," goes on to compare the division into conscious and unconscious to the splitting of consciousness which occurs in double personality, and states that, "if in such a splitting of personality the consciousness remains constantly joined to one of the two conditions, then this is called the conscious mental condition, the one separated from it, the unconscious." Clearly this comparison is not permissible, because the doubling of personality is a phenomenal event capable of being directly observed, while the unconscious of Freud is a conceptual abstraction. Moreover, while it is possible that one dissociated personality may exert some influence upon another, it is obviously not the same order of influence as that which Freud conceives to exist between the unconscious and the conscious.

In Freud's conceptions of the *ego* and the *id*[2] a further division of the mind is formulated, whose relations to the conscious and the unconscious, and to Janet's dissociation, now call for consideration. Freud describes the *ego* as "the connecting organization of the mental processes in an individual[3]," and regards it as centred round the perceptual system of the psychical apparatus. The remainder of the psyche he calls the *id*. The ego is properly a differentiated portion of the id, developed by the influence of the outer world acting through the perceptual system. It endeavours to bring the influence of the outer world to bear upon the processes arising from the id, and to

[1] Hitschmann, *Freud's Theories of the Neuroses*, English translation, New York, 1917, p. 80.
[2] Freud, *Das Ich und das Es*, Wien, 1923.
[3] *Ibid.* p. 14.

replace the pleasure-principle, which reigns without restraint in the id, by the reality-principle. Perception plays in it the part which falls to instinctual force in the id[1].

It does not require demonstration that the division into ego and id is a division of a conceptual and not of a phenomenal kind, and one therefore which has no direct relation to the division formulated by Janet. The demarcation between the ego and the id, moreover, cuts the psyche in a plane entirely different from that in which the demarcation between conscious and unconscious is conceived. This difference is, indeed, expressly emphasised by Freud, and he points out that, while consciousness (and the foreconscious) are entirely confined to the ego, and while the id is entirely unconscious, yet the ego is also in part unconscious. The carving of the psyche along these various conceptual planes is of course a quite justifiable performance, provided it satisfies the demands of scientific utility. The concepts which Freud has fashioned, however, seem to have a fluidity and plasticity which, although no doubt remarkably convenient from the point of view of adapting them to the clinical phenomena observed, make their incorporation in a consistent and intelligible theory a matter of considerable difficulty.

The various characters assigned to the ego, for example, are so disparate in kind as to make the conception of the ego blurred and elusive. These characters are in part topographical, in part dynamic, in part of a conceptual order, and in part of a phenomenal order. The ego is in the first place the co-ordinating organisation of the mind, to which various dynamic functions are also ascribed; then it is the part of the psyche differentiated by the influence of the outer world, and it is also the channel and the controlling agent of the processes passing between the psyche and the outer world; it can be an agent directing the activities of the organism, and it can also be an

[1] Freud, *Das Ich und das Es*, Wien, 1923, p. 27.

object on which the libidinous desires emanating from the id can be directed. Dr Jones has remarked of the super-ego, "How can we conceive of the same institution as being both an object that presents itself to the *id* to be loved instead of the parents, and as an active force criticising the *ego*[1]?" and a similar difficulty would seem to arise in reconciling the manifold aspects assigned to the ego. No doubt the word "ego" can be used in relation to all these manifold aspects, but is it always the same thing to which reference is being made? The ego as a co-ordinating organisation of the mind is a clearly cut conception, but is an organisation of this kind really compatible with the notion of the ego as the portion of the psyche acting as the channel between the psyche and the outer world? Is it implied that a connecting organisation only appertains to that portion of the psyche which is in relationship with the outer world, and that the id possesses no such organisations, but only a mass of discrete and independent processes?

Consider for a moment the case of double personality described above. It is easy and legitimate to regard the normal personality and the one-fifth man as constituted by a split in the portion of the psyche communicating with the outer world, and to interpret this split as a manifestation of two independent co-ordinating organisations, that is to say, of two egos. But there seems to be evidence of the existence of yet another co-ordinating organisation further in the background, a sort of ego-in-chief, which has engineered the creation of the two independent egos in order to achieve its ends. This ego-in-chief must by definition be a part of the Freudian ego and not of the id, and we must therefore assume that a part of the ego acts in a way which splits another part of the ego into two. We seem here to be in need of Occam's razor, but it is the kind of difficulty which arises when

[1] Ernest Jones, "The Origin and Structure of the Super-ego," *The International Journal of Psycho-analysis*, Oct. 1926.

we endeavour to combine in a single entity a dynamic with a topographical ego.

There is a further meaning of the term "ego." It is used to denote an introspectual immediate apprehension, what the man-in-the-street means by "me." The Freudian ego clearly cannot be wholly identified with this "me," because the former is stated to be in part unconscious, an attribute which is hardly applicable to an introspectual entity, but it may perhaps be suspected that the introspectual "me" is the paste which binds together the various disparate concepts included in the Freudian ego.

These criticisms upon the fascinating speculations of *Das Ich und das Es* will serve to indicate the difficulty experienced when we endeavour to envisage, from the standpoint of methodology, the extraordinarily fluid and plastic concepts which Freud employs. Freud's work has been carried out along the road of clinical observation, and he has made and modified his concepts as he went along. It is to this circumstance that the fluidity and plasticity are presumably to be ascribed. The modification of concepts in the light of further facts of observation is of course an unimpeachable proceeding, but it carries with it the possibility that the concepts may ultimately have ascribed to them a complex mass of attributes which do not easily hang together. Such a characterisation, while it facilitates the fitting of the observed facts into the theories, inevitably blurs the precision and definition of the latter, a serious defect when we are dealing with a system of conceptual constructions.

We have taken up the position that these various conceptual constructions of Freud lie on an entirely different methodological plane from the classification of phenomena which constitutes Janet's dissociation, and that confusion of thought inevitably results unless the distinction of plane is rigidly observed. This distinction of plane becomes of importance when we examine one of the very few references which Freud makes to the problem of multiple personality. In *Das Ich und das Es*[1] he states that the ego may be the subject of various identifications, and that, if these identifications are unusually strong and incompatible with one another, a splitting of the ego may occur; he then hazards the conjecture that the secret of cases of multiple personality may be that each of the various identifications alternately draws consciousness to itself. Now Freud also holds that the super-ego arises as an identification performed by the ego, an identification which presumably is regarded as of the same order as those other identifications capable of producing a splitting of the ego. It is true that he emphasises the peculiarity inhering in the super-ego, but he attributes this to the circumstance that it is the first of the identifications of the ego, and that it is the heir of the Oedipus complex, and thus incorporates in itself objects of unrivalled importance[2]. But surely the distinction is more fundamental than this, and depends in the first place on the entire difference of plane existing between a conceptual abstraction and an observed phenomenon. Apart from this it would be theoretically possible for the super-ego to appear as a dissociated personality, a supposition which is clearly inadmissible.

If we leave the phenomenal plane on which the dissociations of double personality are observed, and move to the conceptual plane where we may legitimately seek a dynamic explanation of the phenomena, the concepts which Freud has constructed become of undoubted utility. Were it not that the inquiry would take us beyond the limits of this paper, it would be interesting to consider the bearing of these concepts upon the phenomena observed in the case of double personality described above. How are we to explain, for example, the genesis of the one-fifth man? Clearly this personality arose as an expression of resistance to the resuscitation of repressed material. It always appeared whenever such resuscita-

[1] p. 35.   [2] *Ibid.* p. 60.

tion was attempted, and was always characterised by a blank ignorance and denial of everything which had previously been resuscitated. On the other hand, it was equally characterised by its crystallisation round myself, and its intense hostility to me. Yet in the course of the investigation this hostility was temporarily transferred completely to another individual, the one-fifth man preserving its character as a resistance to resuscitation, but with its hostility to me changed into entire friendliness. How can all this be related to Freud's hypothesis of identification? Clearly this and other similar problems are stimulating and attractive, but they cannot be examined here, nor indeed at all without a preliminary lengthy description of the clinical details of the case. These considerations impel us to reflect, however, upon the remarkable absence of double personality from the literature of psychoanalysis. Not only are the references to the subject scanty in the extreme, and case material conspicuously wanting, but there is little evidence of even an interest in the peculiar problems which these phenomena involve. It will perhaps be profitable to speculate upon the causes underlying these striking circumstances.

To begin with, it may be contended that double personality is an artificial affair. The one-fifth man, for example, was clearly an artefact developed in the course of the patient's treatment, and it cannot be gainsaid that most of the cases of multiple personality described in the literature have undergone an extensive growth under the influence of the hypnotic methods of investigation employed. Such growth is hardly likely to occur under the method of psychoanalysis. But it cannot be seriously maintained that all examples of multiple personality possess this artificial character, and, even if they did, they would not be less worthy objects of serious study.

Moreover, it is not merely that psychoanalysts are not interested in multiple personalities; they make practically no use whatever of the conception of dissociation, of which multiple personality is only the most striking instance. The real issue is not therefore the relation of psychoanalysis to multiple personality, but its relation to the phenomena of dissociation in general. Explanation here would seem to take us once again into the sphere of methodology. The psychoanalyst has a line of approach altogether different from that followed by the investigators of multiple personality. The accent of his interest is not on the manifestations observed on the phenomenal plane, but on the dynamic factors conceived to lie behind them. The conflicting forces on this latter plane are the things that matter, and whether they manifest themselves on the phenomenal plane as one or other of various possible symptoms, or whether they lead to the complete splitting of double personality, is of comparatively minor importance.

Kardiner[1], in a recent review from the psychoanalytical standpoint of McDougall's *Outline of Abnormal Psychology*, describes the line pursued by Freud in these words. "Not only did a clinical entity, like a phobia, have certain descriptive phenomena, a morphology, a history of psychological antecedents; it had also a *dynamism and mobility*. The symptom, its phenomena and antecedents, were relegated to a position of secondary importance, according as it became evident that these phenomena represented the disease process to a very limited degree only. The symptom was observed to take on protean forms, varying with circumstances, but also to remain in contact with certain living forces and conditions. The symptom, from a psychological point of view, became less and less circumscribed, was seen to have a large number of antecedents and determinants, and was kept alive by an *instinctive drive*, whose gratification was thwarted by a group of internal and external factors." Again, "He (McDougall) laments that Freud never uses

[1] Kardiner, "McDougall's Compromise with Psychoanalysis," *Mental Hygiene*, July 1926, p. 536.

the words dissociation and disintegration in the sense in which they are used by Morton Prince and Janet. The difference lies here. Repression is the name of an active, living, and purposeful process; the success that it has varies. Where it fails, the repressed material returns in another form, the symptoms. The symptom, therefore, appears to be 'dissociated,' and to have an independent existence. One can use the word dissociated to designate the return of repressed material; but we know that what appears detached from the aims and purposes of the individual is still a living part of him. Thus the word dissociated is well to use in a descriptive sense, but not in a dynamic[1]."

Kardiner attributes the divergence of the schools of Janet and Freud to "the fundamental difference of methodology between a descriptive psychiatry, whose aim stops with explanations, and a dynamic psychiatry, whose purpose it is to reconstruct the methods of nature[2]." This view emphasises the distinction of plane which has been insisted upon in this paper, although its interpretation of the nature of that distinction is certainly not the same.

It may be said, however, that even if the symptom, with its phenomena and antecedents, be relegated to a position of secondary importance, it still preserves some degree of importance. Its form and relationships on the phenomenal plane are not devoid of interest, and on that plane dissociation is an obvious fact. We can sympathise with the psychoanalyst when he states that he cannot incorporate Janet's methodology into the method of psychoanalysis, but we should like to obtain from him a dynamic interpretation of the facts which Janet and others of his school have observed, and among those facts the phenomena of dissociation and of double personality are surely worthy of note.

[1] Kardiner, *op. cit.* p. 528.   [2] *Ibid.* p. 511.

INDEX

Printed in the United States
By Bookmasters